The Health of a Rural County

Perspectives and Problems

The Health of a Rural County

Perspectives and Problems

Editors and Primary Authors

Richard C. Reynolds, M.D.
Sam A. Banks, Ph.D.
Alice H. Murphree, M.A.

A University of Florida Book

The University Presses of Florida
Gainesville / 1976

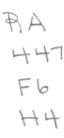

Library of Congress Cataloging in Publication Data
Main entry under title:

The Health of a rural county.

"A University of Florida book."
Bibliography: p.
1. Rural health services—Florida—Lafayette Co.
2. Community health services—Florida—Lafayette
Co. 3. Medical education—Florida—Lafayette Co.
4. Lafayette Co., Fla.—Rural conditions.
I. Reynolds, Richard C., 1929–   II. Banks,
Sam A., 1928–   III. Murphree, Alice H.,
1921–
RA447. F6H4   362.1′09759′816   75–35753
ISBN 0–8130–0525–6

TYPOGRAPHY BY CANON GRAPHICS
TALLAHASSEE, FLORIDA

PRINTED BY THE ROSE PRINTING COMPANY, INCORPORATED
TALLAHASSEE, FLORIDA

Contributors

Sam A. Banks, Ph.D., formerly Associate Professor in the Department of Community Health and Family Medicine, College of Medicine, and in the Department of Religion, College of Arts and Sciences, University of Florida, is currently President of Dickinson College, Carlisle, Pennsylvania.

Leighton E. Cluff, M.D., is Professor and Chairman of the Department of Medicine in the College of Medicine, University of Florida.

Margaret B. DiCanio, Ph.D., is Assistant Professor in the Department of Sociology, Memphis State University, Memphis, Tennessee.

Richard A. Henry, M.D., is Professor in the Department of Community Health and Family Medicine, College of Medicine, University of Florida.

Alice H. Murphree, M.A., is Associate in the Department of Community Health and Family Medicine, College of Medicine, and Associate in the Department of Anthropology, College of Arts and Sciences, University of Florida.

June Remillet, R.N., M.A., is Director of Public Health Nursing at Florida State University and was formerly Director, Division of Public Health Nursing, College of Nursing, University of Florida.

Richard C. Reynolds, M.D., is Professor and Chairman, Department of Community Health and Family Medicine, College of Medicine, University of Florida, and also Acting Public Health Officer, Lafayette County.

Emanuel Suter, M.D., is Director, Division of International Medical Education, Association of American Medical Colleges, Washington, D.C.

George J. Warheit, Ph.D., is Professor in the Department of Sociology, College of Arts and Sciences, and in the Department of Psychiatry, College of Medicine, University of Florida.

Contents

Foreword

BASIC HEALTH SERVICES for rural populations are a concern of health planners throughout the world. Solutions are sought for settings ranging from relative economic and technologic abundance to extensive poverty. Regardless of the prevailing level of development, however, rural life differs from its urban counterpart. Sparse population, low levels of personal income, poor communication, incomplete governmental infrastructures, and depressed educational opportunities are only a few of the troubling factors which characterize rural settings and intensify the problems accompanying the shortage of health care personnel. Unfortunately, advances in biomedical and clinical sciences, together with accompanying technological developments, have accentuated a disparate situation between rural and urban environments. A knowledgeable but disappointed public has developed a greater awareness of deficiencies in health services provided for certain segments of the population; in the United States, this cultural-technical dichotomy has produced a critical lack of confidence in the medical profession.

Unable to eschew some measure of public accountability for health, medical schools have been drawn into the community care setting. With increasing frequency, appropriations by state legislatures and the United States Congress for medical education are being linked to responsibilities for providing primary care physicians and health care services in certain areas. These internal and external pressures have directed the attention of medical faculties to the distribution and quality of services being rendered by their graduates, and many faculty members are taking a close look at their academic programs and accomplishments in this respect. They recognize that the educational process has relied too heavily on the care provided in referral hospitals. Consequently, in the mind of the student, illness has been accorded an entity which is independent of the ill patient. Because students acquire professional behavior and skills in a setting which separates the patient and illness from the normal living environment, the young physicians later seek a similar insulated health environment for their professional activities.

This cause and effect relationship between the educational setting of clinical learning and the malaise in medical care services throughout the country (and the world) has not always willingly been recognized by teaching hospital faculties. Nevertheless, medical schools have begun to seek service affiliations which could add a new dimension to their educational milieu. With the exception of the well-known preceptorship program under general practitioners, many community medicine programs do not lend themselves easily to educational designs. As a result, some medical schools have developed their own community programs, predominantly in urban but also in rural settings.

These programs are challenges for medical school faculties whose scientists may have little or no experience in community-based activities. The need for competency in disciplines not usually considered basic to the practice of medicine, such as sociology, cultural anthropology, systems engineering, economics, and the like, has necessitated additions to the faculty. Curricular adjustments often are needed as well, in order to allocate the time necessary for a community medicine clerkship and the sciences basic to it. These changes cause stressful situations in medical schools; as a result, even a successful program in community medicine may face obstacles within as well as outside the institution.

The story which unfolds in this volume, however, is one of a successful establishment of a community health program by a medical school. Initiated and established by Dr. Richard C. Reynolds in a rural community in Florida, this community health program has become an integral part of the academic milieu of the University of Florida College of Medicine. It is respected both by faculty and students, while serving an indispensable role in the lives of those in Mayo and in Lafayette County.

Having had the privilege of observing and occasionally assisting in the development of this endeavor, I should like to list a few key factors, seemingly critical for its initial as well as for its continuing success:

In 1964, long before a specific project was planned, the College of Medicine reviewed the entire educational curriculum. Faculty opinion revealed a need for adding a dimension of medical activity different from that being offered by the university hospital. It was defined only vaguely at that time as "community medicine"; several years of subsequent debates readied the faculty for undertaking the Lafayette County program.

Mrs. Alice Murphree, as a member of the Division of Behavioral Sciences of the Department of Psychiatry, conducted a study of rural life in Lafayette County, an area where there was no physician or organized medical care. Her original study served as a base line for several new studies and programs of evaluation.

Despite a declining economy and population, Lafayette County enjoyed unusually progressive leadership and did everything possible to promote the establishment of this program.

Participation of several medical school and university departments was important. Of critical importance proved to be the interest of the chairman of the Department of Medicine in developing an outreach program suitable for educating students, house staff, and faculty. The Department of Medicine was willing to support a community-based activity at the expense of many other demands for development.

Equally as significant was the willingness of the county and medical school to finance the project jointly from their own resources without requesting federal assistance. Only later were grant funds received from private foundations (Commonwealth, Carnegie Corporation, and the Robert Wood Johnson Foundation).

Finally the program had the good fortune to have a director with personal and professional qualifications ideally suited for its development.

All of these factors helped to overcome resistance and assure success. During its first five years, this program (as well as others initiated by the Department of Community Health and Family Medicine) has gained general acceptance by academic and community peer groups.

It becomes evident from this volume that community health or community medicine is a composite of various disciplines and inter-woven activities. It involves the knowledge and skills necessary to provide services needed to preserve health, prevent illness, and cure disease. It requires that an individual be treated in the context of the total family and community environment. Community medicine must have its foundations in clinical medicine and public health, blending them into an integrative discipline. It does not aim to make a community medicine specialist of an undergraduate medical student, but rather to impress upon him or her the interaction between individuals and their environment and the importance of this interaction in terms of health and disease.

There is little doubt that the Lafayette County community medicine project can serve as a model for others in this country and abroad. While providing basic health services to a total population, it also affords access to high quality specialty services. It considers the population as a whole and promotes its general well-being; and it affords students an opportunity to perform within a community set-ting while still under faculty supervision.

EMANUEL SUTER, M.D.

Introduction

MEDICAL SCHOOLS throughout this country during the past decade have initiated many community health clinics. The common objectives of these health care projects have been to provide some health services to citizens often isolated for various reasons from ordinary medical care and to develop educational settings in communities that would complement those of the university teaching hospital. The reasons for establishing these community health projects have included the interest of some medical educators in orienting their schools toward an understanding of the problems of ambulatory health care, desire to train personnel responsive to the needs of such care, altruism, social consciousness on the part of some students and faculty, and opportunistic probings by the medical school for a larger patient constituency to serve the needs of the teaching hospital.

The Lafayette County Health Center at Mayo, Florida, reflects, in part, all of these ambitions. It has been and continues to be successful in providing health services to the citizens of the county. It has been even more successful in altering the character of one medical institution, by directing the attention of some of its faculty and students to the medical problems of ambulatory health care and the influences of family and community character in their identification and resolution.

The inhabitants of this one rural county probably differ little from the people living in many other similar rural counties in the United States. The descriptions of their jobs, incomes, attitudes, values, and health probably vary little from those of most rural citizens in this country. In depicting a specific county in some detail, the authors have tried to make it possible to examine the health problems of a broader rural constituency.

The genesis of this book resulted from the activities of the University of Florida Colleges of Medicine and Nursing in the establishment of the Lafayette County Health Center in Mayo, Florida. The Health Center, for obvious reasons, was quickly dubbed the "Mayo Clinic." Two years after its opening, a professor of medicine in Florida, in trying to reach the renowned Mayo Clinic in Rochester, Minnesota, asked the local operator to place a call to the Mayo Clinic; the response was, "Which one?" This may be an apocryphal story but it represents the rapid acceptance of this small rural health center into the milieu of the University of Florida College of Medicine.

On opening day, January 6, 1969, the Lafayette County Health Center had 17 patients. By the end of the first year, 5,488 patients had visited the clinic; by the end of the second year, all but a few of the county's residents had been to the new clinic at least once. Within the first five years of operation, more than 32,000 patients had visited the clinic, physicians had made 1,700 house calls, public health nurses had made 2,300 home visits, and approximately 1,800 x-rays had been taken. The clinical content and procedures involved in this rural practice are reported in more detail in Chapter III.

Since the first day, there have been continuing efforts to provide new and better health services for the county. An expanded school health program, the monthly *Health Letter,* the weekly services of a clinical psychologist and of a pediatrician, a new emergency room, even a weight-watchers' program illustrate some of these ventures.

During the first five years, there were times when the clinic meant the difference between life and death for some of the people in the county. More often, the clinic meant the difference between a long trip to receive medical attention and having excellent medical care near at hand. Several times a patient would have required hospitalization had the clinic staff and equipment not been available in Lafayette County. For a great many county residents, it meant continuing peace of mind just to know that the clinic was there, if needed. Certainly, many people have continued to receive at reasonable costs regular health care not otherwise available to them.

The first five years of operation also have added a significant dimension to medical and nursing education at the University of Florida. Two hundred ninety-three medical students and 109 nursing students have lived and worked in Lafayette County during some portion of their educational careers. In addition, six medical students came from other universities to work in Lafayette County, including four from Panama, one from Scotland, and one from the University of Pennsylvania. Sixty-two residents in medicine, twelve residents in ophthalmology, and four in nursing also had the opportunity to experience, at the community level, the intricacies of meeting health needs as perceived by the community. The great majority of all personnel involved have expressed a real appreciation for the experience; already some of the young physicians and nurses are seriously considering practice in rural areas.

This clinic has now been in continuous operation for nearly six years. A large share of credit belongs to the citizens of Lafayette County. The combined wisdom of the members of the original Community Advisory Committee tempered the plans of the medical school faculty. The committee clearly interpreted the moods and attitudes of the people of this rural community for the health professionals. The committee explained to the county residents the limitations of the clinic, such as the need for rotating resident physicians and, therefore, the impossibility of having their "own" physicians, and the impracticality of delivering babies at home or at the local health center. Presently the Community Advisory Committee is being replaced by a Lafayette County Health Trust, a group of seven citizens appointed by the county commissioners and empowered with the responsibility for health planning and administration of all health affairs in the county. Faculty members from the Colleges of Medicine and Nursing favor this arrangement and look forward to the maturation of this unique governance for county health affairs.

The Lafayette County Health Center represents various groups—local citizens, the University of Florida faculty and students, employees of the Florida Division of Health—cooperating to provide health care and working toward the resolution of rural health problems. This book tries to capture the experiences, the studies, the efforts of these people in their concern for the health of the citizens of one rural county.

There is one author in this book who tries to catalog the character of illnesses brought to the clinic by the inhabitants of this rural county. The list of diseases, however, does not begin to describe their health problems. Fortunately, in this study doctors have been joined by people trained in psychology, sociology, and anthropology.

Health is not limited to a description of people's ailments and what doctors did to relieve them. Health is seen as a state of mind, a set of expectations and attitudes differing for men and women and old and young, black and white and rich and poor.

Many edited volumes are "nonbooks," compilations of vaguely related rewritten articles. This undoubtedly will be a criticism of this book. What shared concerns, however, do give coherence to this work? The contributors focus on a common target from various conceptual angles. The people of Lafayette County and the concern for their health provide the bond that brings these health professionals and social scientists together. The experienced past and anticipated future of these rural citizens and the educational goals of the J. Hillis Miller Health Center of the University of Florida have served to fashion the framework of health care and the content of this book.

Several chapters (II, IV, VI, VII, and VIII) stress the importance of understanding the matrix of customs, attitudes, and expectations among rural health care recipients. To be effective, physicians and other health personnel must recognize the existence and significance of consumer values even when attempting to alter such attitudes. Similarly, the introductory chapter indicates that health planners should be cognizant of the tenacious, long-term needs of rural populations. Likewise, health educators should recognize the need to incorporate, in the curriculum and experiences of health professionals, an understanding of such concepts and attitudes toward health held by various groups of people. These challenges are not of recent vintage, and their lengthy history must be understood if care is to be effective.

In like fashion, some chapters (II, IV, and X) emphasize the complexity of existing communication patterns and the difficulties that health personnel unacquainted with rural culture may encounter. Similarly (Chapters VI, VII), rural consumers' health attitudes, expressions, and behaviors cannot be understood apart from the economic, educational, and social influences embedded in rural life. Rural America is a community, a web of enduring, closely related political, religious, and family systems that mold all attempts to better rural health.

The authors' attention to the past has been matched by a growing sense of imminent challenges on the health care and health education scenes, demanding new approaches and imaginative planning. The contributing physicians agree that a new health system is a necessity for effective rural care, but they are uncertain as to what that system should be. New personnel and structures, new educational programs are required. In Chapter V, a creative response is described: incorporation of the physician's assistant into the medical community. Chapter X adds that, in the rural setting, traditional functions of medical care must be expanded to include emphasis upon health education for the consumer and upon identification and prevention of health problems. The chapter on nursing education (XI) points to the formative effect of experiences in rural health care upon the basic goals and self-understanding of students in the health professions. Each author seems to be saying that, in the struggle for better rural care, the health professionals themselves can be transformed into more effective agents.

Each author echoes the knowledge that old ways and new demands posed by rural communities will require thoughtful reevaluation and planning and rigorous action. Shallow solutions and hasty assessments will not suffice. The section "Studies in Rural Health" suggests the need for better ways of judging the effects of health care procedures on the well-being of a community and methods of measuring the impact of community structures on the success and limitations of rural health systems.

Books published by university presses often present studies of a subject from the viewpoint of a singular discipline. The editors are well aware that a sociologist or an economist or an anthropologist would focus more sharply and in greater depth on selected aspects of the health problems in a rural county. It is said, although we are not in agreement, that a scholar does not study Europe. He studies the economies or political science or sociology of a certain period in European history. The purpose, of course, is to pursue knowledge in greater depth. Survey courses in colleges are seldom the teaching responsibilities of scholars. In similar ways, medical and nursing education has become increasingly the responsibility of specialists. Although medical research and the care of the very sick have benefited from the ever increasing fractionation of health care, an understanding of the health problems and needs of society members appears to have lessened.

The Health of a Rural County is a study in breadth. It is not all encompassing, but its authors try to deal with some issues concerning the health of the residents of one small rural county in north Florida.

Its authors represent varied disciplines. From different stances they have reviewed selected problems of rural health care. The results are sometimes uneven, but it is hoped that they will provide the reader with a better understanding of rural health.

RICHARD C. REYNOLDS, M.D.
SAM A. BANKS, PH.D.
ALICE A. MURPHREE, M.A.

Rural Health and a Rural County

THIS SECTION HIGHLIGHTS the distinctive aspects of a rural society and the effect of these sociocultural characteristics on its citizens' health and care. The focus of the book is on the knowledge derived from one county's attempts to solve its health problems. The significance of these findings for current issues in national health care delivery is considered.

The first author indicates the impact of rural poverty, population trends, and social structure on the health of the people. The higher incidence of illness, accidents, death, and psychosocial impairment in rural settings, the difficulties in obtaining health manpower, and the relatively low utilization of health facilities are described. The chapter concludes with an analysis of the potential resources and opportunities for effective health care to be found in rural settings.

A portrait of the settlement, development, and present state of Lafayette County, Florida, is offered in the second chapter. This author traces the development of industry, housing, and the religious, educational, and recreational functions in this rural community. A detailed description is given of past and present health care facilities and health seeking patterns. The chapter closes with consideration of the effect of the media, church, schools, and political structures on the community's health care patterns.

I. Rural America and Health Care
A Brief Perspective

Richard C. Reynolds, M.D.

RURAL AMERICA includes people living on farms or in nonfarm communities of less than 2,500 residents. Altogether 55 million people in the United States live in rural areas; this number of rural Americans has remained essentially stable for the past five decades.

The geography of rural America is as varied as the mountains of Maine, the hollows of Appalachia, the plantation communities of the South, and the prairies of the Midwest. Common features are sparse population, low family income, poor schools, and an inadequate to almost nonexistent health care system. A few rural counties, because of unusual agricultural success or proximity to urban areas, do not characteristically suffer all the usual rural problems.

Although rural America is often considered an agrarian society, increasingly fewer rural residents are occupied with farming. The mechanization of agriculture has reduced rapidly the number of farmers, and various government policies have reduced the acreage in production. In 1920 three-fifths of the rural population were farm workers. By 1970 only one-fifth of rural citizens worked on farms.

For the most part, industry has bypassed rural regions and located near urban or suburban communities, where there are a greater variety and number of employee resources. Unemployment in rural America is not common but underemployment and low salaries are characteristic. One notable exception occurs among the

5

miners in Appalachia. The miners, whose job skills are often limited to mining itself, remain after the mines close, resulting in a high incidence of unemployment for this particular region of rural America.

The population of the rural United States is made up predominantly of children and older adults. The young adult and the middle-aged person often leave their rural homes because of few job opportunities. The loss of these vital and energetic age groups contributes to the apparent apathy of many rural towns.

People do leave their rural homes for the city. Those who remain, however, comprise a stable population at odds with the current mobility of the people of the United States. Vance Packard in a recent book, *A Nation of Strangers,* states that the average American family will move fourteen times. Approximately 18.5 percent of the total population of the United States moves annually and 7 percent actually move to another county. This exaggerated population mobility is not characteristic of many rural towns. In Mayo, Florida (population 750), five surnames represent 20 percent of the listings in the telephone directory.

Another example of the relative stability of rural Florida's population is Gilchrist County with 3,500 residents. The Department of Sociology of the University of Florida repeated a survey, made one year earlier, of one-third of the households of Gilchrist County and was able to interview 95 percent of the original respondents.

The stability of the rural population is also reflected in a rigid social structure. Compared to urban communities, the rural family unit is more cohesive, divorce may be less common, and motivation among rural high school graduates to continue their education in college is not as great. Rural county boards of education favor recruiting teachers who have been reared in their own or similar rural areas. This tends to minimize the introduction of new ideas into the school system and discourages change. In the South, segregation has given way to integrated schools and places of business. The attitudes of segregation persist, however, and most black residents find few job opportunities and even fewer chances for job promotion. The young adult black residents have left en masse for the large city. This trend adds to the complex multiple problems of the inner city.

The church remains a strong focal point of rural social activity. Almost everyone belongs to a church and most churches are small and family-like in their constituency. Religion is predominantly Protestant and nowhere in this country is the work ethic more strongly endorsed.

Change of social customs and habits in rural regions proceeds slowly. In one effort, the faculty and students of the Lafayette County Health Center responded to the wishes and needs of the high school students to develop a program in drug and sex education. The principal refused to permit this program, because he believed that it would be frowned upon by the parents of the students. Experience has shown his judgment to have been correct. Sections of this book contain the results of altering the health care system of one rural county. The catalog of successes and failures could easily apply to other attempts at social change, such as those in education or political structure.

No spectrum of illness is characteristic of rural people. They suffer heart attacks, develop cancers, and are disabled by strokes with the same frequency as people living in metropolitan communities. The apparent tranquility of rural residents is challenged by the increased percentages of suicides and homicides and of individuals with alcohol problems. A look at the mental health of rural people reveals marked psychosocial impairment. There appears to be a direct relationship between psychosocial impairment and the degree of rurality and poverty.

Statistics in themselves never tell specifically who is in the hospital or whose baby has died. Impersonal as they are, they do provide data to describe the overall health of rural people.

Six more infants per thousand births die yearly in rural areas. Automobile accidents are more often fatal in predominantly rural states. In North Dakota and Mississippi, fatal automobile accidents occur at the rates of 63.4 and 70.1 percent, respectively, compared to the rates of 41.8 and 41.7 percent (per 100,000) for New York and Massachusetts. This difference is attributable, in part, to the lack of health facilities and personnel, particularly to the lack of an adequate emergency medical service in most rural regions.

In large metropolitan areas, 9.8 percent of the people have some activity-limiting chronic illness; in rural areas, 16.4 percent have similar illness. Rural males experience 1,710 days of disability per 100 person-years; urban males have only 1,340 disability days per 100 person-years. Restricted activity of males between the ages of forty-five and sixty-five amounts to 2,370 days per 100 person-years for the rural residents and 1,980 for urban citizens.

The same disproportion is present in health manpower and health facilities. The most rural locations have only 50 physicians per 100,000 population; the most urban settings have 150 physicians. The 10 most urban states have more than 50 dentists per 100,000 residents, while the 10 most rural states have fewer than 46. Considering these same states, there is little difference in available hospital beds. The rural states have 3.6 beds and the urban states have 3.9 beds per 1,000 people. The adequate number of hospital beds in most rural locations is the result of the Hill-Burton legislation passed in 1946, which provided financial support for the construction of hospitals. The quality of services, however, is deficient in many rural hospitals. Fewer than 50 percent of the hospital beds in Arkansas and Montana are accredited, but more than 75 percent of the hospital beds in Delaware and Connecticut have been approved by the Joint Commission on Accreditation of Hospitals.

With fewer facilities and health personnel, utilization of health services by rural people is significantly less. They have 25 percent fewer physician visits than urban citizens. Whereas 1,000 urban residents average a total of 901.6 days in a hospital per year, rural people spend only 704.7 days.

Urban families pay an average of $355.00 per year for health services while rural families pay $315.00, despite the fact that all statistics indicate more disability and illness among the rural people. This figure represents not only the limitations of rural incomes which restrict the money available to spend for health care, but also the limited perceptions of these citizens of the health needs that warrant seeking health services.

There is little question that federal fiscal legislative responses to health needs favor the large metropolitan areas. Although the rural population of 55 million is 25 percent of the total population of this country, only one-eighth of Regional Medical Program funds was dispensed to rural locations for improving health care. Similarly, less than 10 percent of federal funds which were used to establish neighborhood health centers throughout the country were used in rural settings.

The federal government is aware of the deficiency of the health services in rural America. The Comprehensive Health Manpower Act of 1971 specifically encourages medical schools to identify and enroll those "individuals whose background and interests make it reasonable to assume that they will engage in the practice of their profession in rural or other areas having a severe shortage of personnel in such health professions." Whether a physician establishes practice in a rural setting results from a complex interaction of his own background, his professional desires, and the peculiar characteristics of the rural community. Evidence indicates that medical students with rural heritages tend to return to similar areas for practice. The acculturation process of college, medical school, and residency usually occurs in a large metropolitan community. This has an impact on some students with rural backgrounds who choose not to return to rural locations to practice. Specialty training, which is accentuated if not overtly encouraged by many medical schools, does not produce the type of general physician most needed in rural areas.

In rural areas, one out of every four persons is poor. This compares to one out of eight in the cities and one out of fifteen in the suburbs. Being poor, however, has many ramifications other than not having available money to spend. It means that housing is often inadequate, the tax base of the rural community is constricted, and the schools suffer from lack of ancillary teaching resources. With a depressed economy, all local social services are decreased and communities become more dependent on state and federal support.

Poverty has a major impact on the individual's perception of his health needs. In 1954 in a small upstate New York village, Koos separated the citizens into classes according to education and income. Table 1, which is adapted from his book, *The Health of Regionville,* shows the difference in understanding between high and low income groups of the need to seek medical care when faced with flagrant medical symptoms. Poverty and low levels of education within any population group act as impediments to health care. The availability of health services is obviously not a simple answer to health care needs of the poor or uneducated. Efforts at improving education and the incomes of the poor rural people must accompany the delivery of health care, if this is to be successful.

There are strengths in rural America as well as weaknesses and deficiencies. Useful value structures of a previous generation are sustained. In a day of "Future Shock," rural communities act as a reservoir of habits and attitudes that at least tend to slow down the rapid changes of society.

A recurrent theme in surveys of rural populations is the high incidence of psychosocial impairment. This is confirmed by a survey done in Lafayette County and described in a subsequent chapter in this book. What remains unexplained is the tolerance of rural communities toward the considerable number of individuals with measurable mental illness. People who might not be able to function in an urban setting are able to live in a rural community outside of an institution. Thoreau wrote that "The mass of men lead lives of quiet desperation." Although rural people have many emotional problems, their lives in rural America do not seem as desperate as those of their city brethren.

TABLE 1

PERCENTAGE OF RESPONDENTS IN EACH SOCIAL CLASS RECOGNIZING
SPECIFIED SYMPTOMS AS NEEDING MEDICAL ATTENTION

Symptom	Class I	Class II	Class III
Continued coughing	77	78	23
Persistent joint and muscle pains	80	47	19
Blood in urine	100	93	69
Excessive vaginal bleeding	92	83	54
Loss of weight	80	56	21
Persistent headaches	80	56	22
Pain in chest	80	51	31
Lump in breast	94	71	44

NOTE: Class I represents people of high income and educational attainment in the community. Class III includes those with minimal incomes, little education, and unskilled jobs. Class II characterizes the middle class of the community.
SOURCE: Adapted from Koos, 1954.

Juvenile delinquency is ubiquitous but much less common in rural communities. In 1964 the rate of delinquency court cases per 1,000 child population was 33.9 in strictly urban areas, 23.6 in semiurban areas, and only 10.6 in rural areas. Perhaps these statistics are somewhat skewed, because rural delinquents are often handled through unofficial channels. Nevertheless, indications are definite that rearing children in a rural setting mitigates delinquency. Past efforts have been aimed largely at changing personalities in order to eliminate delinquency. Today, the theory is that changing the social situation may be more strategic in the prevention or elimination of delinquency. Perhaps rural communities already provide the appropriate social setting for bringing up children with minimal delinquency.

A simplistic solution to urban problems is to reduce the density of city populations by moving people back to the country. The flight of the white middle class to the suburbs may be a trend that will extend into the more rural counties. The disenchantment with crowds, anonymity, traffic, and crime characteristic of urban living is causing some redefinitions of life style by many urban and suburban residents.

II. The Anatomy and Physiology of a Rural County

Alice H. Murphree, M.A.

CONSISTENT WITH THE TITLE of this volume and with this particular chapter, it seems appropriate to introduce the county by using medicine's traditional academic format.

Lafayette County is an approximately one-hundred-year-old, predominantly white, rural county of the South with an age-skewed population. The presenting complaint is a constricted economy and a severely impaired growth rate. Secondary complications have included lack of localized health resources over a prolonged period of time. Several life crises have contributed to the primary complaint. While guarded, the prognosis is somewhat optimistic, particularly with respect to the cited secondary complication. There may be reason to expect that the ongoing treatment of the secondary complication, in the form of the university-sponsored clinic, will contribute to reducing the severity of the primary complaint.

In the following much abbreviated life history and present status of the county, emphasis will be placed on events and relationships pertinent for considering community health and health care delivery. An effort will be made to place the material within the context of the rural setting, particularly in the southeastern United States.

THE SETTING

To consider one small geopolitical division, such as Lafayette County in north Florida, as a discrete entity apart from other times,

12

places, and people is misleading. Such a rural county shares certain life-style aspects with other southern rural areas, with the South generally, and with all other rural sections, but it contrasts sharply with the urban and suburban milieu. Despite the sharp contrast with the urban ghetto, however, a rural area may share similar economic disadvantages and may also be a partial source for the ghetto's dilemmas. Population migration is urban directed and personal phenomena such as attitudes, economic capabilities, and health conditions are simultaneously transportable and tenacious. Many rural problems, transplanted to the cities, become compounded!

On the other hand, north Florida, with several frosts and freezes each winter, also contrasts in many ways with the semitropical remainder of the state. It has neither citrus groves, space centers, nor Disney World. Contemporary, southbound tourists, using ground transportation, pause briefly, if at all; those who fly bypass it.

Historically, north Florida—in which Lafayette County is more or less central—was not settled by the wealthy planters or European aristocrats. It was not part of the stereotypic antebellum South, because the land was marginal for the type of agriculture associated with the plantation system of the South. Although there were extensive landholdings and some slavery, by and large, land was used for timbering. Although limited, the arable land was, and still is, good for pasturage and such crops as watermelons, peanuts, legumes, and predominantly flue-cured tobacco. The bulk of these small farms were settled by northern Europeans, usually of yeoman stock. The land's marginality also accounts for the relatively late settlement pattern in this part of the South, creating a frontier-like aura.

It may be noted that north Florida has much in common with Appalachia. Both, peripheral to the plantation South, were settled by people of similar forebears. Both have constricted economies partially based on extractive activities—mining in Appalachia and timbering, naval stores, pulpwood production, and limited mining in north Florida. Both were divided into small agricultural holdings with some subsistence farming. Both are currently suffering common problems as well—all the concomitant results of restricted economies. The outmigration results in age-skewed residual populations with intricate (almost convolved) kin relationships and, possibly, highly concentrated gene pools. These are significantly stable and homogeneous population groups. Both areas, with many others, suffer multiple health problems and have limited health care.

Lafayette County's dominant topographic features are "the river" (fifty-five miles of the Suwannee River form the northeast border) and "the woods" (cypress ponds and flatwoods to the west and southwest).[1] A strip of high, arable land, varying in width from three to perhaps six miles between "the river" and "the woods," contains the approximately 9,000 acres of cropland and the majority of the population. The bases of the timbering activity are "the woods" and the various acres of agricultural land planted in pine trees as part of the Soil Bank program. The flatwoods section, which contains part of the Steinhatchee Wildlife Management Area, is dotted with lakes, ponds, and creeks. These "woods" are well populated with ranging cattle and hogs as well as a mixed wildlife.

Definition of social and cultural boundaries for the county may be an impossible task. Historically, rural southern people have social and physical origins elsewhere; likewise their contemporary relationships reach to other places and people. For instance, not all its citizens even identify with Lafayette County in all their activities. Many shop, recreate, seek health care, and are employed elsewhere or receive their wages from sources outside the county. Approximately 75 percent of the land is absentee owned. Those living in the periphery, nearer towns other than Mayo, the county seat, identify for various purposes with towns in neighboring counties. For some, such commonplaces as mail delivery or telephone service originate outside the county. Television is ubiquitous, albeit viewed from a distinctive cultural vantage point.

Again, there is also the reality of continuing outmigration. For at least two or three generations, the majority of the young people have been moving to locations with more fertile economic prospects. Many, however, regularly return to visit and a small proportion ultimately return to retire. While acknowledging such relationships in space and time, it is still convenient to consider Lafayette County as a discrete entity. It will be within that framework that the following discussion is set.

Lafayette, with 553 square miles, ranks thirteenth from the smallest of Florida counties. It was not always thus, however: originally, the county had 1,263 square miles; in 1921, a geopolitical division allocated 710 square miles to form Dixie County. In 1890, the first census showed Lafayette with a population of 3,686, and in 1910

1. "The woods" is a large flatwood portion of the county, comprising swamps, cypress ponds, lakes, and heavily wooded areas.

a peak of 6,710 was reached. The population decline, begun prior to the creation of Dixie County, continued, so that by 1970 the figure had fallen to 2,892. Of this latest number, 330 were black. Table 1 gives the census breakdown by age, sex, and race.

The decade between 1910 and 1920 was obviously a crucial one for the county. During that era, approximately five physicians, two dentists, and twelve schools were reported existent in the county. Although some of the physicians were employed by the lumbering companies and the majority of the schools boasted only one room, these figures suggest a much more vigorous economy than has been experienced in later years. Although it was never a big cotton producing area, when the boll weevil struck during that decade, it may have contributed to the initial constricting trend in the agricultural economy. It is suggested that the political division into two counties originated in a land use disagreement between turpentine interests and the cattle growers. Landowners have always been people of power in rural areas.

Interestingly, Dixie County, originally the southern part of Lafayette County, did not experience a comparable agricultural depression and consequent population shrinkage. Dixie showed 6,419 in the 1930 census and a peak of 7,018 in 1940; a sharp drop to 3,928 occurred in 1950, but a renewed growth trend produced 4,479 in 1960 and 5,480 in 1970.

During the early part of this century, then, Lafayette was not the relatively isolated, sluggish, little county that it is currently. It was an integral part of the bustling economic, social, and political center of the state. Two significant factors combined to create population shifts. First, technological innovations reduced labor requirements. Second, the timbering interests utilized a much larger labor force to produce naval stores than is required in contemporary pulpwood production. As the timbering labor market declined, the turpentine workers, mostly blacks, sought employment elsewhere. There were no ties to keep them—they had never been among the landowners, not even of small farms, and agriculture also was experiencing reduced labor requirements.

Subsequently, each generation saw the bulk of its youthful vigor leave the county for the same reasons. Except for helping one's parents on the farm or in the few small town businesses, job opportunities are extremely limited. Ironically, the population flow patterns account for the fact that unemployment approaches non-

TABLE 1

1970 POPULATION, LAFAYETTE COUNTY, BY AGE, RACE, AND SEX

		All Races		White		Negro	
	Total	Male	Female	Male	Female	Male	Female
All ages	2,892	1,444	1,448	1,269	1,293	175	155
Under 5 years	256	132	124	105	108	27	16
5 – 19 years	842	430	412	398	342	82	70
20 – 39 years	630	319	311	285	278	24	33
40 – 64 years and over	775	385	390	355	363	29	27
65 years	389	178	211	165	202	13	9
Median age	30.4	29.5	31.5	31.6	33.9	15.1	17.0

SOURCE: U.S. Department of Commerce, Bureau of the Census, 1970, p. 164.

existence. The limited number of newcomers are usually retirees, not productive young people. There is much truth in the commonly repeated lament, "There just ain't nothin' here for young folks."

The major sources of livelihood in the county are still agriculture and forestry. The farming produces tobacco, dairy products, beef cattle, hogs, broiler chickens, and small grains. Many farm operators have full- or part-time employment outside the county. The other major source of livelihood, pulpwood production, is almost entirely absentee owned or controlled. A small group, employed by various local, state, and federal governmental agencies, also operate farms to supplement income. Two small industries, not locally owned, are a pleasure-craft boat factory, which employs approximately forty to fifty people, and a concrete block plant, which has a maximum payroll of fifteen. The most prestigious jobs are those with regular payrolls, i.e., in the school system, the various state and federal agricultural and transportation agencies, local government, and the pulpwood companies. Table 2 gives the data on family and individual income, and Table 3 depicts those with less than poverty level income.

The one town, Mayo, had a population of 687 in 1970. There is a small hamlet (Day) with a post office, two stores, and three churches providing a nucleus around which approximately two hundred people cluster. Several other locally recognized places are identified by the predominant church, crossroads store, or topographical feature. Running roughly southeast and northwest across the northern part of the county is U.S. highway 27, and a state paved road runs south from Suwannee County through "the woods" to the Gulf of Mexico. There are several paved farm-to-market roads in the agricultural part of the county and many well-graded dirt roads. A short railroad spur into the northern section of the county is all that remains of an original accessibility to both freight and passenger service.

With one or two exceptions, all housing is of single unit design, although more than one family may occupy a given house. Construction ranges from the small, simple, rural frame house to the most modern middle-class brick or concrete block dwelling, with all the contemporary appointments and appliances. In addition, there is an increasing prevalence of mobile homes varying in size from one bedroom with no bath to three bedrooms with two baths. Although only a limited number of the modern homes are visible from the main highways, more can be seen along the county roads.

The typical old rural southern house is of unpainted heart-of-pine

TABLE 2

INCOME FOR FAMILIES (N = 755) AND
UNRELATED INDIVIDUALS (N = 219), 1969

Median family income	$5,368
Median income for unrelated individuals	$1,260
Per capita income	$1,978
Mean family income (by source)	
Wage or salary	$5,780
Farm self-employment	$5,019
Social security	$1,381
Public assistance or public welfare	$ 681

SOURCE: U.S. Department of Commerce, Bureau of the Census, 1970, p. 507.

boards with two, three, or more rooms. The house is usually divided by the "dog trot" (an open-ended, six- or eight-foot-wide hallway running the depth of the house)—the coolest place in the house in summer. Front and back porches are common and the structure is raised at least a foot off the ground on bricks, rocks, or posts. The kitchen may be detached, accessible by walkways from the back porch. The pitched roof is of wooden shingles or tin and, in older homes, is often moss covered. If the windows are without glass, solid wooden shutters are protection against cold and insects.

A later type of construction, locally termed a "boxed" house, omits the "dog trot" and porches and has glazed windows. The external joints between vertical pine boards are covered with one-inch strips, and the elevation from the ground is retained. The interior is usually ceiled with wall- or plasterboard, but, again, often neither interior nor exterior is painted.

TABLE 3

PERCENTAGES OF INCOME AT LESS THAN
POVERTY LEVEL

Income less than poverty level	
Percent of all families	23.8
Percent of all persons	30.5
Percent of persons 65 years and over	23.6
Percent of all households	45.8

SOURCE: U.S. Department of Commerce, Bureau of the Census, 1970, p. 507.

A type of wooden house built about forty years ago often contains two or more bedrooms, a separate dining room, a kitchen, and a living room. Still elevated from the ground, the houses have painted clapboard outside walls, porches, glazing, screening, interior partitions of plaster, and asbestos shingle or tin pitched roofs. Most houses of this latter type are in town. A more modern variation is the shell house, produced and sold nationwide. When new, these are screened and neatly painted externally, but the interior is left for the purchaser to partition and paint.

A significant dimension in the social setting of a community is recreation. Here, church functions, along with school activities, make up the major forms of group social activity. Both adults and children have a keen interest in all school athletic events, and participation in sports is often mentioned as an attribute. Other school functions such as plays, trips, meetings, and projects are also forms of group recreation.

There are various church-connected associations for men, women, and children. Reference is frequently made to one's Sunday school class or to choir rehearsal or the deacon's meeting. There are home demonstration clubs and sewing circles, and the Masons, Eastern Star, and Shriners have small but active memberships.

Hunting is a primary source of recreation for men and boys and, occasionally, for women. Many families maintain hunting camps in "the woods" and spend varying periods of time there during the specified hunting seasons. Young boys do much target practice with BB guns or 22-caliber rifles and join hunting groups as early as ten or twelve years of age.

Almost universally, both men and women are enthusiastic about fishing, but usually men fish together and women fish together, not in couples as do urban residents. It is common to see two or more men driving toward "the river" or one of the lakes with poles tied to the car or pulling a boat on a trailer. It is equally common to see people sitting on the bank of a pond, lake, or creek, bait can beside them, fishing with a long "cane" (bamboo) pole. Often women go fishing after morning household chores are completed or early in the afternoon when the "dinner things are cleared way." Some of the hunting and fishing, particularly fishing, probably has economic value.

There are other, less popular, water-oriented recreational activities. Several crystal clear, fresh water springs, situated in the flood plain of "the river," provide swimming opportunities. "The river" and some larger lakes are water skiing sites for a small but growing number of enthusiasts. Interestingly, however, many rural people cannot swim and express strong fear of drowning.

A very important form of recreation is "visiting" among family and friends. "Visits" occur primarily in daylight hours and consist of long conversations about local events, both past and current, which ramble from topic to topic as time permits. Both men and women enjoy this pastime, with men more often remaining out-of-doors and women sitting on the porch or indoors. This practice is so prevalent that one is on very serious business indeed if he does not stop and "talk some" for at least five minutes when he meets a friend or kinsman. To refuse to "visit" is to invite suspicion or condemnation for rudeness.

A final aspect of the setting is the tempo of daily life. On a typical, early spring, weekday morning, the residents of Lafayette County, like other rural people, are early risers. Immediately after breakfast, various vehicles begin moving—agricultural equipment goes to the fields, the school buses start rolling on their rounds, a few cars or pickup trucks head for out-of-county employment destinations, and others go to town or to "the river." Among the earliest businesses to open are gas stations. Here, the pulpwood trucks "gas up" and the "crews" congregate to ride to the woods.

By 8:30, school has "taken in," stores and offices are open in town, wash begins to appear on clotheslines and back yard fences, and the tractors have made visible progress in the fields. There is somewhat of a midmorning lull in household activity until time to prepare dinner—the noonday and main meal in most homes. In Mayo, things move rather slowly, with a slight flurry at "coffee time" as people go to the cafe or drugstore. As the courthouse clock slowly starts to strike twelve, however, doors can be heard slamming all over town; and by the twelfth stroke, car engines are started and most people are on their way home to dinner. Stores and offices reopen at 1:00 P.M. and the leisurely pace resumes.

At 3:00 in the afternoon, when school "lets out," the tempo in town and in the county again picks up. School buses start their return trips, the town children are seen walking to the drugstore or to after-school jobs, while others "set about" their chores at home. At five o'clock, offices in town close, the crews are returning from the woods, last minute grocery shopping is completed, and by six o'clock the only businesses open are the convenience store, gas stations, cafe, motel, and restaurant. By 8:30, the only lights in town are street lights, those at the 7-11, or at the clinic, signaling an emergency. Along the highways traffic has all but stopped, lights in the houses have begun to go out; the automatically lit chicken houses and the isolated dusk-to-dawn floodlights at various farms make bright spots in the otherwise dark county.

HEALTH CARE RESOURCES

In 1969, the University of Florida College of Medicine established the teaching clinic in Mayo. For the ten years prior to that, formal health care resources indigenous to the county had been extremely limited. There had never been a hospital. The one practicing physician had retired and the last dentist had never been succeeded. In the Public Health Department, there were one full-time public health nurse, a part-time sanitarian, a public health officer two half-days a week, and a full-time secretary-clerk. The pharmacy was owned and operated by a licensed pharmacist. There were two practicing licensed midwives, supervised by the public health nurse. The county had hired a veterinarian and also owned and operated an ambulance. The less than half a dozen registered nurses or nurses' aides were all practicing outside the county.

Representation of the other helping public agencies was similarly sparse. The state welfare social worker spent one day a week in the county. Vocational Rehabilitation and Crippled Children's Commission counselors were available locally about once a month. There were no local mental health workers. As a result, often the county judge and sheriff were forced to act as health intermediaries without benefit of appropriate professional advice.

Customarily when illness occurred, it was tentatively diagnosed within the family, and the mother made the ultimate decision regarding care. She drew on her own as well as kin's and neighbors' accumulated experience, and often an accepted self-treatment remedy was used. This latter might range from a conjure through old-timey remedies to patent medicines. The second step would be consultation with one of the "nurses" when she got home from work or a visit to the drugstore to see what "Doc" could suggest. If the symptoms disappeared at any point in this process, the illness was considered cured. If the symptoms did not respond to the treatment, usually medical help was sought from a physician. If the illness seemed sufficiently serious, simultaneously with any of the steps, healing reinforcement would probably be requested from the church.

The decision to go to the doctor was not taken lightly. A visit to the nearest physician involved a round trip of approximately 45 miles plus the heavily weighted aspects of cost and time. In addition, there was the element of transportation itself. Not everyone owned a vehicle and neighbors, family, or even the sheriff might be called upon. Often, for one reason or another, the nearer physicians were not the choice, and the trip could be as much as 100 or 150 miles. Frequently, prescriptions were filled in the town where the physician practiced. Obviously, the same conditions prevailed for dental visits or hospitalizations.

Despite generalized positive statements concerning the 'family doctor," research results indicate that often he would not have been visited for many years. Regular check-ups for the entire family were rare. In one pre-clinic study involving families of eighth-grade school children, only four of the seventy families reported such preventive measures, and 79 percent saw a physician only for a sufficiently tenacious specific complaint. The same study also revealed that only 13 percent of the children and 27 percent of the households had regular dental examinations.

The community tends to assume responsibility for the care of its incapacitated members. It is common for family and neighbors to "pitch in and help" when illness strikes or is extended. The women bring food, help with household chores, and participate in patient care. On the farms, the men may contribute to agricultural work, and often the men "set up" all night with someone considered too ill to be left alone. Possibly, the eagerness to accept joint sponsorship with the university for the clinic in Mayo reflects this tendency for the rural community to assume care for its own members.

In the context of health resources, a significant social phenomenon has been observed as contributory to the underutilization, or even absence, of a valuable resource. This involves the presence of "peripheral professionals" in rural areas. They are peripheral in that they do not, or are not permitted to, function at the maximum capabilities expected of their professions, nor are they geographically situated in the professional centers.

Some individual members of the various professions—physicians, attorneys, nurses, teachers, counselors, ministers, and others—are often seen by rural residents as having personal problems. Frequently, the problems result in an addiction of some type or in social behavior deviant from the accepted rural norm. Given the previously discussed interest in local events and the predilection for gossip ("visiting"), all behavior considered aberrant rapidly becomes commonly known. Consequently, the image of the specific professional and the perception of professional standards, including those in the health fields, may become somewhat marred; this, in turn, may result in some hesitation to accept services.

It seems ironic that the population outflow may syphon off the potential indigenous professional resources and that some of the resident professionals who should be among the greatest assets to a rural community are not or, at least, may not be viewed in that light. Many of the much needed talents seem to be located elsewhere. This phenomenon must be considered to affect health and health care, both directly and indirectly.

Patently, the teaching clinic is, by far, the most significant health resource in Lafayette County at present. Excellent ambulatory care is available, at modest fees, twenty-four hours a day, seven days a week. Approximately eight thousand patient visits during 1971 indicate the degree of utilization. There have been indications of the effectiveness of the health education programs originated in the clinic; one of the primary goals, however, to provide comprehensive health care for all county residents, as yet has not been achieved.

It is recognized that the rotation pattern in staffing, required by medical educational parameters, is not the form of health care delivery most acceptable to the rural community. Much preferred is the traditional "ole family doctor" model—the physician intimately familiar with the patient and his family for long periods of time. Maximum possible continuity is strived for by faculty members and through improved record systems, and it is felt that utilization of the clinic, with time, will help alleviate this difficulty.

COMMUNITY INSTITUTIONS AFFECTING HEALTH CARE

Along with education and economic conditions, religion probably most affects health and health attitudes. Religious affiliation is one of the principal elements of identification in the community. Church membership has high value, and whether one is Baptist, Methodist, Church of God, or some other denomination is basic to placement in the social order. That one may be unaffiliated, while rarely admitted, is also highly significant.

In philosophy and value system, Lafayette County fits the Bible Belt pattern. With recognizable pride, community members frequently refer to themselves as "good Christian people" and to their environment as a "good" one in which to raise children. The Southern Baptist churches have the largest membership, the Methodist are next, followed by the various smaller sects such as Church of Christ, Church of God, and Assembly of God. There is a small Episcopal chapel in Mayo with services once or twice monthly, but there are neither Catholic, Presbyterian, nor Jewish groups. The black community of approximately 300 supports four or five small Pentecostal churches.

The belief in a firm relationship between health and religion pervades all denominations. The Church of God and the Assembly of God churches, however, traditionally practice divine healing. At times of illness, the preacher is called to the house for prayers, and the congregation is routinely expected to support his efforts with individual and group prayers. Also, prayers "for the sick," usually identified by name, occupy a prominent place in the regular services. Historically, these congregations did not "believe in doctors" but "trusted in the Lord"; however, contemporary membership may seek medical help as routinely as do others. No matter what the church affiliation, good health is commonly recognized as a "blessing" and illness (along with other misfortunes) is considered punishment or "God's will." Also, a widely expressed belief is that "Doctors can't heal without God's help."

A slightly more obscure effect of religion upon health concerns that rigid moral code, accepted as "ideal" locally, by which, not unexpectedly, not all people consistently live. The overtly accepted nineteenth-century ethic of the Bible Belt includes numerous strict expectations of social behavior. This is combined with the primary, face-to-face, social relationships of a residual population, where everyone knows (or is related to) nearly everyone else. A third significant element in these dynamics is the group introversion and the predilection for gossip. As a result, figuratively, there is a skeleton in every closet—but no doors on the closets! Behavior aberrant to the acknowledged, but not necessarily adhered to, ideal elicits standard rationalizations but must also result in certain degrees of guilt. Such specific tensions between religiously sanctioned ideal and real behavior can be considered to affect, directly, the emotional etiology of disease.

It is also suggested that the rigid social restrictions of the rural southern community may be psychologically analogous to the physical restrictions of an urban ghetto. In this sense, the free life in the country may be mythical! Particularly is this true when one knows his behavior is "wrong" and simultaneously knows the community is watching and aware of his actions. There is little anonymity in the rural community and feelings of paranoia can be based on reality.

Further, the family contributes to the overall health of the community members in ways other than direct health care. It is the locus of primary socialization; here the rigid value system is taught and reinforced. Again contrary to the espoused ethic of the "good Christian" family, however, there is some frequency of broken homes, divorce, desertion, and remarriage. Neither adultery nor illegitimacy is an unheard of (or unnoted) occurrence! These psychological factors relative to family stability are believed also to affect the children's and adults' emotional health.

The psychosocial-religious dynamics discussed above are combined, in an agricultural setting, with a constricted economy and the uncontrollable vagaries of the weather and of markets. Such a situation could, in part, contribute to the incidence of psychosomatic complaints and the tension-based illnesses presented in the clinical setting.

The support, both psychological and otherwise, expressed in some of the family and other social dynamics should not go unnoted, however. The typical person in the rural setting may feel secure in knowing that those people with whom he has almost daily contact are predictable in their responses to him, that those to whom he may turn for assistance need be no cause for anxiety, just as he is well aware to whom certain reciprocal favors or gifts are due. Such formal and informal exchanges, either within the family network or with neighbors and friends, are so commonplace as to suggest their being almost unconscious. Also, where there are few strangers, there is little to fear from the unknown in personal interaction. This element of security in social relations well may be one of the rural communities' greatest strengths.

Another strong relationship is the one between the educational institution and the size and economy of the county. Although top quality education is a sincere aspiration of all concerned, the seriously limited rural resources have ramifications in this, as in other, cultural components. This is expressed in the difficulty that rural high school graduates have in competing for college entrance with graduates of urban or suburban school systems.

The bulk of the population has had at least some high school education, although illiteracy does exist, particularly among older residents. The several schools have been consolidated into one unit, kindergarten through twelfth grade, located in Mayo. A county-sponsored school bus transports college-age students to the community junior college in a neighboring county. For many in Lafayette County, a round-trip school bus ride of forty miles is not new. Again consistent with the value system, particular care is exercised to employ a faculty that adheres to the "good Christian" ethic. The majority of the school personnel were born and reared in the county or a similar rural community—thus enhancing the stability of local values.

Partially because male physical prowess is esteemed in the rural community, school athletic events (particularly football) are well attended and receive relatively strong support from all citizens. A concern for good health practices is implied here. Although health education, per se, has not figured largely in the school curriculum, the Public Health Department has mounted the usual annual immunization and screening programs in the school. These latter have been greatly augmented by the presence of the teaching clinic and the participation of the medical and nursing students and faculty from the university.

Social and civic organizations in the county support various health-oriented projects from time to time. The Rural Development Authority and the Rotary Club have long helped defray health care costs for a limited number of indigents. Various Bible classes and other church organizations may contribute in some way when a member's family has costly health problems. The Mayo Women's Club regularly schedules programs and projects concerning nutrition or health as do the home demonstration clubs. When the teaching clinic was established, the local organizations contributed varying support, primarily with x-ray, ophthalmologic, and laboratory equipment.

The Lafayette County Commission is the basic governing and administrative entity for the county. Each of the five districts elects a commissioner to represent it, and the county also elects a county clerk as secretary for the commission. This body has the responsibility for much of the health sector of the community. The commission budget includes items for building and grounds maintenance of the Public Health Department, the salaries of its personnel, county welfare, and a small allocation for hospitalization of indigents. With recommendations from the State Board of Health, the commissioners also participate in hiring of Health Department personnel as they do representatives of some other state agencies. With the advent of the clinic, which shares the Public Health Department facility, a close, cooperative relationship has existed between the County Commission and the administrative personnel from the university.

An organization with long tenure in rural areas is the Cooperative Extension Service. Each county is served by representatives of the state university system in the positions of county agent and home demonstration agent. Lafayette County is assigned one each. The agents are expected to (and do) live in their respectively assigned counties and function as educators and as information sources from the State Agricultural Experiment Station. The Extension Service has both explicit and implicit programs for health, including instruction in food preparation, nutrition, and home and farm safety.

Finally, in considering the institutions influencing the health of the community, we must include the media. A weekly newspaper, published in Mayo, is devoted primarily to local newsworthy events. It is the vehicle for all public notices, including those of the Public Health Department. Items involving various health projects and programs and other health information also appear periodically. The university clinic personnel have submitted pertinent health articles authored both by staff and students. Also, there is a recently initiated *Health Letter,* mailed monthly from the university clinic to each residence in the county. This carries informational items pertaining to clinic staff and programs as well as articles focused on health education. Local radio stations in neighboring counties are received in Lafayette County as are the television stations in Tallahassee and Jacksonville.

It needs to be emphasized that all media represent the value framework of their originators but may well be viewed from the culturally determined framework of the local recipients. One of the media's most immediately pervasive results is the influence of television commercials, particularly those for patent medicines. Community members often tend to self-diagnose and self-treat in terms of the most current products being advertised. The pharmacist frequently receives requests for new products that have been advertised in, but not delivered to, the local community.

CONCLUSION

This chapter has presented the major pertinent facts concerning Lafayette County in order to facilitate an understanding of the setting in which the University of Florida Colleges of Medicine and Nursing established and maintained a teaching clinic. The health conditions and the available resources prior to the coming of the clinic are discussed, as are many of the cultural components contributing to those conditions. To some extent, the county's location, geographically in space and historically in time, was established.

One of the principal emphases concerns similarities and differences. While Lafayette County is not unique, in that it has shared the vicissitudes common to all rural areas (perhaps more than its share), it is very different from urban and suburban communities. The people are enculturated with the typical rural southern mores and experience the advantages and disadvantages of rural life, both of which contrast sharply with other life-styles and experiences. Significantly, though, given the population flow patterns, the *results* of such enculturation and rural life-style *do* find their way to other settings.

One component of rural life, the constricted economy, strongly affects all others, and Lafayette County, unfortunately, has not escaped these effects. In fact, the possibility exists that ameliorating the economic difficulties will be the key to solving many of the concomitant problems. There have been suggestions (difficult to assess or document) that the presence of the clinic has influenced directly the local economy by improving the local business financial condition. It is anticipated that the continuing presence of the clinic will, with time, improve the health and, indirectly thereby, all other components of social setting in this rural community.

Medical Care of a Rural County

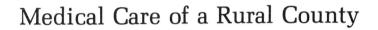

THE CHAPTERS COMPOSING this section deal specifically with actual ongoing attempts to offer medical care to rural residents.

In Chapter III, an overview of past studies of the content of rural medical care is given, along with the results of recent research conducted at the university-sponsored rural health center in Lafayette County. Findings include a profile of the examinations conducted, symptoms described, diagnoses obtained, and medication prescribed for a sizable sample population. In addition, rural patients' perceptions of their overall health and functionality are seen in relation to their use of the clinic.

The following chapter outlines a history of health care in Lafayette County and describes the planning and development of the rural health center. The effects of the private practitioner, the Hill-Burton Act, the Sears Roebuck Foundation program, and the newly created Health Service Corps on rural health care problems are discussed. Suggestions are made for the creation of a more adequate system of health care delivery in the rural setting.

Finally, the problems and satisfactions of the rural general practitioner are presented, including a cross section of the country doctor's day. Establishing the need for new kinds of health personnel in the rural setting, the author reports on the development of an education program for rural physicians' assistants and the effect of such personnel in a pilot project.

III. The Content of Rural Medical Practice

Richard C. Reynolds, M.D.

FEW STUDIES have been done to characterize the content of rural medical practice. In 1970, Steinman reported the prevalence of various illnesses among the residents of a rural county in eastern Kentucky. These data were obtained by screening large samples of the population and did not necessarily represent patient identification of illness significant enough to require medical care. Among these people examined in Appalachia, one-fifth of the infants (less than two years) had otitis media. There was a 30 percent prevalence of respiratory infection among the entire population. Even among children (ages 2–13), disorders of the ears, eyes, and respiratory tract were present in 35, 23, and 13 percent, respectively. Worm infestation probably occurs in more than 50 percent of children in many rural areas.

Last and White studied the habits of care of five different physicians in Vermont during the winter of 1964–65. There were obvious differences in the contents of the individual practices which represented the interest and habits of the individual physicians. Respiratory diseases were the most common conditions treated in all of the practices. Twenty-six percent of all patient visits to these five physicians were for respiratory conditions and the range varied from 20 to 33 percent for the individual practices.

In contrast, the faculty of Johns Hopkins School of Medicine developed in 1969 a comprehensive health care scheme for residents in Columbia, Maryland, a newly built suburban community between Baltimore and Washington. Among the first 9,554 ambulatory visits,

33

19 percent of patients sought treatment for respiratory diseases. In this group, however, 38 percent of the visits were for health assessment or well person care. Perhaps this accent on health maintenance reflects in part the high average family income of $17,000 and the better educational status of this well-to-do community.

The residents of Lafayette County come to the rural health center in Mayo with self-recognized medical problems expecting to understand the nature of their illness, sometimes to obtain emotional support, and most commonly, to find relief from discomfort. The reasons why a patient decides to see any physician or health professional are not clearly understood but represent a sum of individual and cultural behavior patterns, influenced by his immediate symptoms and his concerns for payment of services and the availability and accessibility of the services. The assessment by the patient of the quality and character (ranging from sympathetic, warm understanding to cold, distant, professional) of medical care affects the decision to seek professional attention for a presumed health disorder. This chapter will recount several surveys describing patients who did and did not utilize the health care facilities at Mayo, Florida.

The medical-school- and community-sponsored Lafayette County Health Center represents the only nearby source of ambulatory medical care for county residents. The price is reasonable (five dollars for a routine office visit), and there is a clear understanding among the community members that they will be seen even if they are unable to pay. Since the opening of this health center, some resident from virtually every household in Lafayette County has been treated at the clinic. Actually, more than 95 percent of all the citizens have been seen one or more times. The data presented will represent the utilization of health services by a community. It will minimize the selectivity of patients that any individual doctor has in his practice by virtue of his own peculiarities.

The clinic opened in January 1969. The diagnoses for the first 300 patient visits to the clinic are presented in Table 1. Among these 300 patients, there were only 330 diagnoses established at the time of the first visit. Although the patients were probably questioned and examined in greater detail by senior medical students and medical residents than comparable patients seen in many family physicians' offices, complete histories and physicals were not done on all patients. These diagnoses do summarize the physicians' interpretation of why patients came to the clinic.

TABLE 1

ILLNESSES AMONG FIRST 300 PATIENTS SEEN AT
LAFAYETTE COUNTY
HEALTH CENTER, JANUARY 1969

Acute

Upper respiratory infection, presumably viral	117
Bacterial pharyngitis, sinusitis	35
Gastrointestinal disorders	15
Skin problems	10
Pneumonia	9
Trauma	9
Urinary tract infections	8
Muscular skeletal disorders	7
Other	21
TOTAL	231

Chronic

Hypertension and / or arteriosclerotic cardiovascular disease	29
Chronic lung disease	20
Psychiatric disorders	12
Arthritis	11
Allergy	8
Diabetes	7
Headache	6
Other	14
TOTAL	107

During the months of June through December 1969, 987 patient visits, randomly selected, were reviewed to determine the age, sex, race, and diagnoses of this clinic constituency. The sex and race distributions for these 987 different patients are presented in Table 2.

TABLE 2

SEX AND RACE OF THE INDIVIDUALS
PRESENTING FOR 987 PATIENT VISITS

	Males	Females	TOTAL
White	399	439	838
Black	61	88	149
TOTAL	460	527	987

Of the approximately 2,800 people in Lafayette County, 10 percent are black and 50.7 percent are male. Among those seeking medical care at the rural health center, 15 percent are black and 46.6 percent are male.

Table 3 reveals the utilization of this clinic by age groups. Comparison to census data in 1968, especially prepared for Florida, reveals reasonable correlation between those age groups using the health center and the actual percentage of all citizens in these same age groups. The clinic clientele twenty years of age or younger represented 42.6 percent of all patient visits, while they actually represented only 31 percent of the total county population. Although 41 percent of the population was older than forty years of age, this segment accounted for 38 percent of all the visits.

In Table 4, the 1,076 diagnoses established among the 987 patient visits were recorded. A simplified arbitrary scheme for classification of illness has been devised to present these data. In addition, the data include the numbers of white and black, male and female residents seen at the health center within each category of disorder. Seldom is more than one diagnosis made for each patient visit.

Respiratory disease, which accounts for 25.2 percent of all diagnoses, is by far the most common reason for patients to seek medical assistance. Diseases of the skin were recognized 112 times (10.4 percent) among 987 patients. There were 27 patients with impetigo, all of whom were under age twenty-one. Diseases attributed to the cardiovascular system were noted 97 times. The majority, 82, of these diagnoses were hypertension and arteriosclerotic heart disease.

Included in the category of clinical procedures and/or follow-up visits were suture removal, dressing changes, and brief return visits to ascertain the response to previous treatment.

Eighty-two patients (7.6 percent) presented to the clinic, free of complaint, for some form of physical examination. These included forty-seven routine or annual physical examinations and twenty-three examinations required by schools or colleges.

Although the clinic refers obstetrical patients to a maternal-infant care clinic in another city, among those surveyed were twelve patients in this category and one baby was actually delivered in the clinic.

It is straightforward to tabulate the age, sex, race, and diagnoses of patients seen at any health facility. These data, however, do not characterize the symptomatology of the patients. They ignore the

TABLE 3

SEX AND RACE BY AGE GROUPS FOR 987 PATIENT VISITS

	Male		Female		Percentage of Total
	White	*Black*	*White*	*Black*	
0 – 2 years	29	8	31	9	7.8
3 – 10 years	61	15	80	19	17.7
11 – 20 years	73	12	72	13	17.2
21 – 30 years	39	9	42	11	10.2
31 – 40 years	41	2	35	9	8.8
41 – 50 years	24	1	34	4	6.3
51 – 60 years	35	4	41	7	8.8
61 – 70 years	41	6	52	15	11.5
71 – 80 years	30	1	26	0	5.7
81 – 90 years	16	0	15	0	3.1
91 – 92 years	2	0	5	0	.7
age not recorded	8	3	6	1	1.8
TOTAL	399	61	439	88	

TABLE 4

DIAGNOSES AND / OR PROCEDURES FROM 987 PATIENT VISITS BY SEX AND RACE

Diagnoses: Diseases Related to	Male		Female		Total	Percentage of Total
	White	Black	White	Black		
Eye	22	7	27	5	61	5.6
Upper respiratory tract	105	10	105	11	231	21.4
acute	(41)	(6)	(59)	(4)	(110)	(10.2)
uncomplicated acute	(61)	(4)	(39)	(6)	(110)	(10.2)
complicated chronic	(3)	(0)	(7)	(1)	(11)	(1.0)
Lower respiratory tract	30	0	11	0	41	3.8
acute	(6)	(0)	(3)	(0)	(9)	(.8)
chronic	(24)	(0)	(8)	(0)	(32)	(2.9)
Cardiovascular system	50	2	39	6	97	9.0
acute	(9)	(0)	(6)	(0)	(15)	(1.3)
chronic	(41)	(2)	(33)	(6)	(82)	(7.6)
Gastrointestinal system	17	3	26	5	51	4.7
acute	(14)	(3)	(24)	(5)	(46)	(4.2)
chronic	(3)	(0)	(2)	(0)	(5)	(.4)
Liver, gall bladder	1	0	1	0	2	.1
acute	(1)	(0)	(0)	(0)	(1)	(.09)
chronic	(0)	(0)	(1)	(0)	(1)	(.08)
Endocrine system	5	0	17	4	26	2.4
diabetes	(4)	(0)	(14)	(4)	(22)	(2.0)
thyroid	(1)	(0)	(1)	(0)	(2)	(.2)
menstrual	(0)	(0)	(2)	(0)	(2)	(.2)
Trauma	34	7	14	3	58	5.3
minor	(33)	(7)	(14)	(3)	(57)	(5.2)
major	(1)	(0)	(0)	(0)	(1)	(.09)
Obstetrical problems	0	0	4	8	12	1.1

	A		B		C		D		E		Rate	
Genitourinary disorders			0		14		7		21		1.9	(1.6)
acute	0	(0)		(0)		(13)		(5)		(18)		
chronic	0	(0)		(0)		(1)		(2)		(3)		(.2)
Skin	54		10		35		13		112		10.4	(9.2)
acute		(47)		(7)		(34)		(12)		(100)		
chronic		(6)		(2)		(0)		(1)		(9)		(.8)
allergy		(1)		(1)		(1)		(0)		(3)		(.2)
Mental illness	13		2		44		11		70		6.5	(3.1)
acute, minor		(5)		(0)		(24)		(5)		(34)		(.37)
acute, major		(1)		(0)		(2)		(1)		(4)		(2.9)
chronic, minor		(7)		(2)		(18)		(5)		(32)		(0.0)
chronic, major		(0)		(0)		(0)		(0)		(0)		
Neurological system	3		0		7		0		10		.9	
Musc. / skel. disorders	25		4		23		4		56		5.2	(3.4)
acute		(19)		(3)		(12)		(3)		(37)		
chronic		(6)		(1)		(11)		(1)		(19)		(1.7)
Nutritional illness	4		0		12		1		17		1.5	
Clinical proc. and / or follow-up	50		8		51		3		112		10.4	
Physical examination	26		6		41		9		82		7.6	
Undefined	8		3		5		1		17		1.5	
TOTAL	447		62		476		91		1,076			

skills or examinations required by the attending physician and do not designate the therapeutic reply to the needs of the patient.

During part of the month of November 1969, the information from 284 consecutive patient visits to the Lafayette County Health Center was recorded on a special form (Figure 1). There were no

TABLE 5

PRESENTING SYMPTOMS OF 284 CONSECUTIVE PATIENTS

Pain	44
Chest-6, Abdomen-8, Extremity-16,	
Back-8, Other-8	
No complaints (follow-up or P.E.)	35
Skin rash	30
Cold	29
Other	29
Results of trauma	28
Sore throat	20
Cough	20
Anorexia, nausea, vomiting	15
Headache	14
Diarrhea	11
Difficulty with urination	9
Fever	6
Bleeding	5
Nervousness and / or fatigue	5
Shortness of breath	4
Dizziness	4
Fainting	3
Swelling, edema	3
Swollen lymph nodes	1
Bronchitis	1
Numbness, tingling	1
Weight loss	1

differences in this subgroup in the age, sex, and race composition compared to the larger group already described.

The presenting symptoms of these 284 patients are listed in Table 5. Altogether there were 283 complaints for 249 patients. Thirty-five patients were seen without any specific complaint, either for a check-up or a follow-up visit that had been requested prior to the period of study. Pain (44 patients) and skin rash (30 patients) were the two most common complaints that brought residents of the county to the clinic. Usually patients presented with one complaint. The average was only 1.1 complaint per patient. Questioning would identify other problems, but the data collected were representative of the patients'

FIGURE 1*

PHYSICIAN-PATIENT ENCOUNTER FORM
LAFAYETTE COUNTY HEALTH CENTER,
MAYO, FLORIDA

Age: Sex: M F   Race: W B

Chief Complaint (Reason for coming to clinic):

Physical Examination (Circle appropriate reply):

   Temp.—Not Done   98   99   100   101   102

   BP —Not Done   Record value: _____

Organ Examined:			Abnormal:		Comments:
Skin	yes	no	yes	no	
Eyes	yes	no	yes	no	
Ears	yes	no	yes	no	
Nose, throat, mouth	yes	no	yes	no	
Lymph nodes	yes	no	yes	no	
Lungs	yes	no	yes	no	
Heart	yes	no	yes	no	
Abdomen	yes	no	yes	no	
Genitalia	yes	no	yes	no	
Extremities	yes	no	yes	no	
Neurological	yes	no	yes	no	
Other: (write in)	yes	no	yes	no	

Diagnosis (write in):

Treatment (list drugs):   Symptomatic   Therapeutic   Counsel

Return appointment: yes   no

* This physician-patient encounter form was used by the physician to record the data
from the patient visit. This was done in addition to the regular record keeping.

indication for seeking medical care. Some complaints notable by absence among these 284 patients included constipation, obesity, and palpitations.

A total of 1,234 examinations were performed on the 284 patients for an average of slightly more than 4.3 examining procedures for each patient. The number of times that each examination was per-

TABLE 6

TOTAL EXAMINATIONS PERFORMED ON 284 PATIENTS

Types of Examinations	Number of Examinations
Temperature	149
Lungs	145
Nose, throat, mouth	126
Heart	102
Ears	100
Skin	93
B.P.	86
Extremities	86
Eyes	85
Lymph nodes	74
Abdomen	65
Other	60
Neurological	41
Genitalia	22
TOTAL	1,234

formed is given in Table 6. Recording the temperature of the patient was done most often (149 times), closely followed by examinations of the lungs, upper respiratory passages, skin, and blood pressure.

The diagnostic formulations among these 284 patients did not differ significantly from the larger group of 987. A total of 369 diagnoses were established—1.3 diagnoses per patient visit. A diagnosis of some form of respiratory disease was made 100 times (35 percent). Diagnosis of a skin disorder occurred in 48 patients (17 percent). Most common were acute skin disorders among children, usually impetigo, poison ivy, or insect bites. Together hypertension and coronary artery disease accounted for 43 of the 44 diagnoses of cardiovascular disease. Mental illness was diagnosed in patients as either of minor (26 patients) or major (4 patients) proportion and of an acute (16 patients) or chronic (14 patients) nature. Mental illness was thought to be a significant impairment to the health of 30 different patients, an incidence in excess of 10 percent.

For these 284 patients, 407 drugs were prescribed (types listed in Table 7). Antibiotics were given to 95 patients, including those with skin infections who received topical antibiotics. Analgesics, expec-

TABLE 7

TYPES OF DRUGS PRESCRIBED FOR 284 PATIENTS

Antibiotic	95
No drugs	50
Other	47
Analgesic	45
Expectorants	36
Tranquilizers—sedative	31
Digitalis	22
Antihistamines	22
Bronchodilators	18
Diuretics	14
Hypoglycemic agent—oral	7
Antihypertensives	5
Oral contraceptive	4
Antihelminthic	4
Hypoglycemic agent	2
Anti-Parkinson	2
Antispasmodic	2
Steroids	1
TOTAL	407

torants, tranquilizers, and sedatives were dispensed less than half as frequently as antibiotics. Fifty patients (18 percent) received no drugs.

In view of these data, two profiles emerge. First there is a profile of patients seeking medical care. Some of these data are presented in Tables 2, 3, and 5. In addition, a profile of the physicians' response to these patients is revealed also in Tables 4, 6, and 7.

Altogether, some type of respiratory infection accounts for anywhere from 25 to 33 percent of all patient visits. Minor trauma, health maintenance concerned with the management of chronic ills such as hypertension and arthritis, and patient symptomatology, requiring only the reassurance that serious illness is not present, comprise other significant causes for patient visits to physicians. This definition of professional talent and skill required to serve most of the rural residents' needs for primary care has resulted in speculation that someone other than a physician could provide such care.

To explore this possibility another rural health care project by the Department of Community Health and Family Medicine in an adjacent county has utilized physician assistants as the primary purveyors of ambulatory health care. This experiment in rural health care is described briefly in Chapter V.

Not any of the data, however, characterizes the health of the rural community members outside the purview of the clinic. What percent of the rural population is not able to function or perform its expected daily tasks, and does the utilization or availability of medical services influence this ability? In an effort to answer these questions, 10 percent of the households in Lafayette County, randomly selected, were identified. A questionnaire was devised to collect brief health data on each member of the household for the preceding week. Each household was interviewed once weekly.

The questionnaire was structured to enable the rural residents to interpret their abilities to perform the daily chores of living. For a wife this might include doing her housework. For a husband it would indicate his usual performance at work. A student would be expected to attend school and participate in the usual activities. All ages were included.

In Table 8, a portion of the data is recorded for the month of March 1970. As defined by the patient, there is evidence of increasing disability with age. Women consistently reported greater disability than men during all the months in which data were collected. The estimate of disability of the members of any household was usually supplied by the female head of the household.

Table 9 contains, by percentages, similar data on disability collected during a five-month period, November 1969 through March 1970. Unfortunately, there are no explanations for the monthly differences that are readily apparent between the "well" and "felt sick, went on" groups. Overall, approximately 10 percent of this rural population characterized itself as not feeling well but still plugging along. Another chapter in this book depicts a high degree of mental health impairment, as measured by the responses of residents from this same county to psychological tests. Perhaps this sense of not feeling well suggests the somatic reflection of psychological illness.

For the months of March, April, and May 1970, the data were reviewed to determine whether the people who claimed disability

TABLE 8

Self-Determined Disability of Rural Residents in Lafayette County

	Men's Ages					Women's Ages				
	0–4	5–14	15–29	30–59	60–	0–4	5–14	15–29	30–59	60–
No. of days well	53	188	77	226	131	35	161	166	227	164
No. of days sick, went on	0	5	7	11	21	0	7	0	39	40
No. of days bed, self-care	0	2	0	1	2	0	0	1	7	6
No. of days bed, with care	3	1	0	0	0	0	0	1	7	6
No. of days in hospital	0	0	0	0	0	0	0	0	0	0

NOTE: Disability is defined by residents interviewed weekly during the month of March 1970 in Lafayette County. Total Days: 1,585.

TABLE 9

Percentage of Disability Days among a 10 Percent Sample of Residents of Lafayette County

	November	December	January	February	March
Well	90.2%	87.6%	95.5%	90.6%	83.9%
Felt sick, went on	9.5	10.4	4.0	7.9	15.9
Bed, self-care	.2	.9	.32	1.3	.011
Bed, with care	.1	.6	.06	.2	.006
Hospital	—	.5	.06	—	.0005

NOTE: Disability is defined by patients interviewed in Lafayette County, during 1969 and 1970. Numbers represent the percentage of days during each month with varying disability.

TABLE 10

PERCEPTION OF HEALTH STATUS AND UTILIZATION OF MEDICAL SERVICES

	Well	Sick, Went on	Bed, Self-Care	Bed, with Care	Hospital
March					
Users (98)	72.4%	17.4%	9.3%	1.0%	—
Nonusers (1,652)	86.9%	11.9%	1.1%	—	.1%
April					
Users (119)	73.1%	20.2%	—	—	—
Nonusers (1,617)	94.7%	5.2%	.1%	—	—
May					
Users (56)	80.3%	19.7%	—	—	—
Nonusers (722)	98.9%	1.0%	.1%	—	—

NOTE: Disability is defined by patients interviewed weekly during March-May, 1970. Clinic users are defined as anyone who went to the clinic for any purpose during the month. (A nonuser one month might become a user the next month.) Numbers in parentheses represent the total patient days.

used the clinic more frequently. In Table 10, the data derived from weekly interviews of members from the selected households are presented, comparing the differences in utilization of the clinic according to the individual's perception of his health status. Obviously the population seeking medical services at the clinic does perceive itself as not feeling as well as the nonusers. This remains a subjective evaluation, however, and there is no evidence from these data that the clinic user is measurably sicker. In fact, both groups, the clinic user and the nonuser, gave similar responses to a list of symptoms. There is still no evidence from the available data that the presence and utilization of the medical services from the rural clinic actually improve the health of the people, measured objectively (morbidity and mortality statistics) or subjectively.

A significant portion of rural medical practice is concerned with the symptomatic treatment of minor illness. Many patient visits to seek medical service are professionally unnecessary, in that the illnesses are often brief and self-limiting. If the patient had a better understanding of the natural course of common illnesses, conceivably he could improve his judgment as to when to seek a physician's services. A bit of circumstantial evidence acquired in Mayo suggests that it is possible to instruct the citizens of a community about illnesses in such a fashion as to change their utilization of the rural clinic.

During February of 1969, an epidemic of mumps occurred among the residents of Lafayette County. From one to three young patients a day were seen at the health center with characteristic swelling of one or both parotid glands. By history and observation, the diagnosis was affirmed and symptomatic treatment prescribed. A medical student working at the clinic prepared the following article on mumps which appeared in the *Mayo Free Press*.

From the *Mayo Free Press*
February 13, 1969

Today's article will cover a very common illness, the mumps.
What is mumps? Mumps is usually taken to mean the very painful swelling of the glands surrounding your ears, known as the parotid glands, and is caused by a virus. There is one gland on each side of the face, and although both sides are usually involved, only one side may be attacked by this virus. If this happens, the person has mumps just the same. Mumps most

commonly affects children between the ages of 5 and 10, although it can affect all ages, including adults.

Can other glands be affected? Yes. Other glands of the body can be swollen with or without the parotid glands being swollen. This includes the pancreas, the coverings of the brain and the male testes or sex glands. However, it is uncommon for these organs to be affected.

Can a man become sterile from mumps? Males before puberty do not run the risk of having their sex glands affected, but after puberty some doctors estimate that up to ten percent of males who get mumps may get swelling of one sex gland. However, it is almost unheard of for a male to become sterile from this, and so he can continue having as many children as he wishes.

Once a person gets the mumps, can he get it again? No. Having the mumps means you have a particular virus, and this virus causes the body to develop its own protection, or immunity, that lasts a lifetime.

Can a person have this immunity without ever having the swollen glands? Oddly enough, yes. For reasons we don't understand, many persons can have the virus—and hence develop lifetime immunity—without ever getting swollen glands or becoming sick. In fact for every three people exposed to the mumps two may get swelling and the third be immune. This is why many adults do not catch the mumps from their children, even though they themselves never remember having it.

What is the treatment for mumps? Today we have no treatment, and the person must wait until the illness runs its course. This lasts usually from four to seven days. He should stay at home and rest. Simple measures like giving aspirin for pain and fixing of soups in place of solid food are frequently helpful, also.

Should a child with mumps be isolated? Mumps is a communicable disease, which means that people catch it from one another. However, doctors have recently found that it probably does no good to isolate a child from his family once he has the swelling. He should be kept from school for the duration of his illness, however.

Is there a vaccine for the mumps? Within the past year a vaccine has become available to protect the people from the mumps, but it has not yet become widely used.

Following this article, patients with mumps visiting the clinic abruptly declined to near zero. The epidemic did continue for several more weeks and an occasional man with mumps orchitis was seen in the clinic.

Virtually every word of this weekly newspaper is read by residents of the county. This brief article on mumps attempted to describe the illness and emphasize that there was no specific therapy. Perhaps it did assist the readers in recognizing the illness and understanding what to do about it. Apparently it resulted in a reduction in the number of visits to the clinic of people with mumps.

During a flu epidemic one fall, the clinic was seeing, daily, several patients with influenza. Usually they would seek professional advice 24–48 hours after onset of symptoms. Another article was prepared for the *Mayo Free Press,* describing influenza and specifically focusing on the complications of this illness among the elderly and chronically ill. Again, the medical students and residents were impressed with a reduction in the number of patients seen early with uncomplicated influenza. Occasional patients with bacterial infections following this viral infection continued to require medical service.

These anecdotal episodes do suggest that health information and education may quickly influence the decisions of patients to seek medical care. Recently the Lafayette County Health Center has begun to publish a monthly health newsletter which is mailed to every household in the county. It regularly includes brief articles on common health problems that are troubling citizens of the rural community. Recent newsletters have reported on tetanus immunizations, impetigo, pesticides, and alcoholism.

The content of rural medical practice in Lafayette County probably differs little from other rural communities in the United States. The data presented here reflect the perceived needs of an entire rural community for medical services rather than an individual doctor's practice, which often is influenced by the traits of the physician. Brief health education efforts may also influence the decisions of patients to seek health care. Illness and disability of the citizenry of a community are only partially reflected, however, by cataloguing the people and the illnesses for which they seek medical services.

IV. Changing Patterns of Rural Health Care

Richard C. Reynolds, M.D.

PRIOR TO THE OPENING of the Lafayette County Health Center, there had been no practicing physician in the county for ten years. The last physician to practice in Mayo, Florida, the county seat of Lafayette County, still lived in Mayo. He had practiced until he was seventy, retired, and, with increasing years, had become feeble and withdrawn from most social contact. Still, he remained remembered and appreciated by the citizens and was the model of physician and the mode of health care that the community identified as best for them.

Although there was no physician active in Lafayette County, there were established patterns of health care. The county health department, a unit of the Florida State Division of Health, operated with one public health nurse, one clerk, and an itinerant county health officer who spent two mornings each week in Mayo. A sanitarian was available for one day a week. Although he lived in Lafayette County, he was assigned to a larger, nearby county for four days each week. His duties were primarily to oversee the possible public health hazards on dairy farms, in eating places, and of septic tanks and water supplies.

Funds to support the county health department were derived from both the county and the state. This meant that the employees of the county health department were responsible to two separate administrative units, which, at times, was confusing. The local people understood that the public health nurse's primary responsibility was to make home visits to the chronically ill or to troubled families. The nursing supervisors at the state level were not indifferent to home visits but wanted the public health nurse to concentrate part of her efforts on a school health program and community health education. Needless to say, the public health nurse was usually recruited locally and tended to heed the wishes of the county commissioners. The county health officer, whose contract specified that he spend 20 percent of his time in Lafayette County, accomplished this through his two mornings each week. He took care of the administrative chores of the unit and for approximately two hours would see patients. It was more or less understood in the community that these clinics were for the poor people, particularly the local black population, who could not be expected to seek health care otherwise. Some members of the community would attend the clinics, however, because of convenience or to take care of routine health problems such as blood tests for various licenses or insurance physical exams.

There is one drugstore in Mayo, Florida, and the pharmacist-owner is often sought for counsel on health problems. Over the counter medicines are discussed and purchased by virtually all the residents at some time. The pharmacist is characteristically called "Doc" by everyone, clearly designating him as a purveyor of health care.

Obviously, the people, by necessity, did seek medical care outside the county. Suwannee County to the north had 15,500 residents served by four general practitioners, all of whose offices were in the county seat, twenty-five miles north of Mayo. These physicians, as the population-physician ratio suggests, were extremely overworked. Located in Suwannee County is a small eighty-bed accredited hospital, which manifests all of the problems of trying to maintain a sophisticated health care institution in a rural region. When a faculty member from the university met with the four doctors during one of their monthly hospital staff meetings, he found a very cool reception. The intent of the medical school becoming involved in the actual delivery of health care to a community was questioned; need for more health care for the people of Lafayette County was denied; even the slight possibility of economic threat to them was posed. Subsequently, the state medical society initiated review of the project, and eventually did endorse this educational and service program.

To the west of Lafayette County is Taylor County with 14,000 residents, seven physicians, and a small hospital. The physicians worked in Perry, Florida, thirty miles from Mayo, and included one surgeon and one obstetrician. When apprised of the university joining with the citizens of Lafayette County to provide some medical services, they were strongly supportive of the idea. They offered their help and counsel, were interested in meeting with the medical students regularly and, as time permitted, in sharing their experiences and knowledge of practice with them. Their support of the clinic did much to offset the concerns of the councils of the state medical society, due to the objections of the other group of physicians.

Dixie County with 5,500 residents is south of Lafayette County. It was served by one osteopathic physician who admittedly could scarcely begin to respond to the demands for his services. He was grateful for any medical help that could conceivably lessen those demands. As an osteopath, he appeared uncertain in his relations to a group of university physicians, but this eased with time. Another rural county, Gilchrist, east of Lafayette, has 3,500 residents, and at the time of the opening of Lafayette County Health Center had one physician who was planning to leave practice (and did) for training in obstetrics.

The citizens of Lafayette County visited the doctors in Suwannee and Taylor counties for medical services. The doctors, for the most part, did not adhere to appointment schedules. The people would drive to the doctor's office and often wait for several hours before they were seen. Frequently friends and neighbors would ride along and spend the day shopping in these communities, which had more stores than Mayo. Some charged to drive the patients to the doctor's office. Five dollars was the usual fare and this was shared by all the riders. Transportation was a problem, because most families had only one car or pick-up truck, and this was commonly used by the male head of the household to get to and from work.

It is difficult to estimate the incidence of untreated acute illnesses or the lack of maintenance health care in Lafayette County. Undoubtedly, it was considerable. During the first year of operation of the Lafayette County Health Center, a public health nursing student studied the fourth-, fifth-, and sixth-grade school children's habits of going to the dentist. None of the black children and only 50 percent of the white school children had ever been to a private dentist. Some of the black children had had dental surveys through the use of a mobile dental unit provided by the Florida State Division of Health. The same questionnaire was given to students in an elementary school in Gainesville, Florida, the site of the university. Over 98 percent of them had been to the dentist and 50 percent within the prior six months. The paucity of dental services obtained by those of Lafayette County is probably illustrative of the fewer health services of all kinds received by these people.

The priority given health care by any community varies according to its perceived needs, particularly in relation to the competing fields of education, roads, housing, and job opportunities. When the clinic was in the planning stages, the county commissioners made a commitment to contribute $8,000 a year to its operation. Recently, as the clinic has come closer to self-support, this appropriation has been reduced to $5,000. To encourage a veterinarian to establish a practice in Lafayette County, the county commissioners were willing to underwrite his support to $12,000 yearly. The veterinarian, whose talents also were needed, served fewer than two dozen farmers.

The role of folk medicine in this rural community is discussed in another chapter. Suffice it to say here that the greater the isolation of the community from organized health care, the more common is the tendency toward folk practice. Changes in communication, particularly television, have homogenized many former culture variations. Concepts of health care are no exception. Folk descriptions of medicine are increasingly the parodies of television advertisements.

The university faculty met with community representatives in early September 1968. The clinic opened on January 6, 1969. Although this represented too brief a period for detailed analyses and surveys of the expectations of community members for health care, several recurrent themes were voiced by the citizens. They wanted their own doctor, preferably a middle-aged, married man of rural southern background. They assumed he would be Protestant. They envisioned their doctor as kind and considerate and available. They understood that no one would always be present in the community, twenty-four hours a day and seven days a week. They assumed or hoped that illness requiring immediate attention would not occur when the doctor was not available. They were explicit that he should provide medical care on a fee-for-service basis. They were proud that they, as a community, paid their bills and that any doctor settling in this county would have a more than adequate income. A brief glance at the economic indicators of this county might challenge the availability of resources for the majority of citizens to purchase any quantity of health service, but this was not recognized by them.

The initial dialogues between representatives from the community and university established that the university was unable to provide a scheme of health care similar to that identified and desired by the community. The university members stated that they could only provide health services as an integral part of their educational mission. They proposed that senior medical and public health nursing students live in Mayo for three to five weeks under the immediate supervision of senior assistant residents in medicine who would change each month. Faculty from the Colleges of Medicine and Nursing would be at the clinic several days a week to provide continuity and supervision and to conduct some classes. All the clerical help would be recruited from the local community. The scheduled clinic hours would be negotiated with the citizens of Mayo, but needed medical services would be available around the clock. The eagerness of the community to have available a nearly full gamut of ambulatory health services facilitated the acceptance of this proposal.

In 1968, the county health department building had been constructed with the aid of federal funds obtained under Hill-Harris legislation. The building was used only by the public health nurse, a clerk, and the part-time county health officer and sanitarian. The structure included three fully equipped examining rooms, ample waiting room, office space, and a conference room. Unquestionably, this was an ideal place to house the proposed clinic. Because of the dual relationship of the county health department with local county commissioners and the State Division of Health, the proprietorship of the building was unclear. The local commissioners offered the use of the building to the university to establish the clinic.

Faculty members then met with the public health nurse, the county health officer, and representatives from the headquarters of the State Division of Health in Jacksonville. The public health nurse was helpful, supportive of the proposed clinic, and knowledgeable about the community. Married to a Methodist minister, she was preparing to leave Mayo as her husband had been transferred to another church. The county health officer was cordial but uncertain of his exact relationship to the students and faculty. Actually, his significant contribution to the health of the county was to conduct his medical clinics two mornings a week; the need for these clinics would be usurped by the new clinic, making this role of the county health officer of little need.

When the concept of the university attempting to provide health services was proposed to the deputy director of the State Division of Health, he was encouraging and supportive and has remained so. A few months after the clinic opened, the local county health officer resigned to return to private practice. When the university proposed to the State Division of Health the functional amalgamation of these two health care units in Lafayette County, the state responded by appointing the faculty member of the Department of Medicine in charge of the university's operation as the acting county health officer. The deputy director of the State Division of Health also was agreeable to structuring the county health department budget to serve best the citizens of the county. In addition, he arranged for some faculty members from the university to meet all the division chiefs of the Division of Health. With time, there have been questions and controversy between those responsible for the clinic and the supervisors from the Division of Health, but at no time has there been unwillingness to address these problems and try to resolve them, always in favor of the citizens of Lafayette County.

Following some initial meetings between the community representatives and university faculty, an advisory council was established. A group of interested self-appointed citizens was to help the university members understand the expectations of the local community and, conversely, to enable the faculty to explain to them the restraints of the university in meeting all their desires for health care. The initial Community Advisory Council included the county judge, a county commissioner, the managers of two businesses, a farmer, and the principal of the black elementary school. (This school was closed two years later and the principal subsequently moved out of the county.) The Advisory Council met with two or three of the university faculty every two to four weeks for six months. At first the council was unsophisticated regarding health care affairs and would quickly and unanimously acquiesce to any suggestions presented by the faculty from the university. The council was helpful in working out the clinic hours, arranging a fair fee schedule, and finding housing for the medical and nursing students and residents. It was hesitant to challenge or contradict any requests or suggestions from the university members, as it did not wish to do anything to block the reality of having available, for the first time in ten years, medical care in the community.

The council did ask whether we planned to deliver babies at the clinic, and whether the university would like the county to try to establish its own hospital. Both of these requests were unrealistic but did represent the views of the local people. It is sometimes a problem to travel 20–30 miles to have a baby. Many also would prefer hospitalization near their home and families and care by their friends and neighbors.

Actually, it took one year before the Community Advisory Council developed a meaningful dialogue with the university faculty. By then, several of the members had begun to understand the educational effort of the clinic, the problems and necessity of personnel rotations, the difficulty of fiscal solvency, and the problems of introducing black medical and nursing students into this traditionally segregated community. The council was able to teach the university faculty the differences between professional definitions of health care needs and the expectations of the community members for health care. As the council became more learned about health care and more comfortable in its role, it became more assertive in its requests. The university members had begun to question the need for night clinic hours. Usually only a few people came, several of whom could have attended the clinic during the day. But even when presented with data which mitigated against the continuation of night clinic hours, the council responded definitely in favor of continuation, and the evening hours were not changed. It also contributed a scheme for collection of bad debts from patients who had neglected payment for medical services. The council has continued its important role as a liaison between the health professionals and the county commissioners and citizens of Lafayette County.

In discussing the changing patterns of health care in a small rural community, it is necessary to attempt to understand why previous methods of health care failed. The former system of health care had centered on a solo general practitioner who had valiantly attempted to meet the needs of the citizens. He worked incredibly hard, knew the foibles of his patients, and, at a time when the value of medical care was largely symptomatic and supportive, provided ample sympathy and understanding for many. This type of physician is becoming an extinct species.

The decline of general practitioners in rural areas can be reviewed by probing the community, the personal, and the professional difficulties. The typical rural community includes from 1,000 to 8,000 people. It may support from one to more than ten physicians, depending on its commercial drawing area. Actually, the total number of people in rural America remains unchanged (55 million for the last three decades). The recent rapid growth of this country has taken place largely in the suburbs. Most residents of small rural communities exist near poverty levels. They have conservative views on education and often hesitate to make the financial contribution necessary for a first-rate public school system. The social activities are strongly family and church oriented. Families are large and often interrelated through marriage. (In Mayo, Florida, five names account for 20 percent of the telephone listings.) Although outsiders to the community are received graciously, there is a long waiting period before they are fully accepted. To the wife of a young physician, this is occasionally a traumatic period. The wife and children of the physician lose identity and anonymity, usually being referred to as Doctor ———'s wife or child. Hunting and fishing and rabid interest in high school sports are major male diversions. A young physician who has spent four years in college, four years in medical school in an urban setting, and further training in a metropolitan hospital is usually not prepared for the social and cultural milieu of a rural community. His wife's expectations from practice usually do not include residence in a rural community. What are viewed as educational limitations for the children will impede a physician's family from settling in rural America. There are, of course, exceptions to these statements. Doctors who have been reared in small communities do return to these or similar locations more commonly than their urban counterparts.

Although community limitations and personal dissatisfactions lead to reluctance to make a commitment to a rural practice, the major reason for not doing so is probably professional dissatisfaction. A doctor, from the first day he enters medical school, associates with other students or physicians. He is involved in a continuous professional dialogue. He becomes used to sharing his medical problems with others and the resulting exhilarations and disappointments that follow the successes and failures in medical practice. In most private practices, there is a decrease in this professional intercourse among physicians, but this loss is accentuated in the rural communities because of fewer physicians and the demanding workload. This intellectual loneliness deters doctors from practice in rural communities.

The refinements of medical care, accelerated as a result of biomedical research, have emphasized the need for specialization.

Medical education is, for the most part, the responsibility of medical specialists. A student tends naturally to emulate and follow his teachers' interests in selection of a medical career. Rural medical practice has fewer opportunities for the supporting structures necessary for specialty practice. The subsequent decline in the training of general practitioners has reduced the number of physicians available for rural practice. Practice in rural localities is rigorous. A doctor is totally immersed in the health problems of his small community. Sixty- to eighty-hour work weeks are common. Doctors are, however, members of a large society that is seeking and getting shorter work weeks. Doctors are not unaware of the twenty-four-hour work week of electricians. Hospitals have little difficulty recruiting emergency room physicians, emphasizing the attractiveness of a scheduled forty-hour work week. This societal change in attitude toward work will affect the practice habits of physicians.

Rural communities need health services yet seem to be in the process of rapidly losing what physician services they do have. The expectation of rural citizens is to recapture the types of services to which they have been accustomed. Personal and professional pressures on physicians entering practice tend to preclude their location in the country.

In recent years, there have been several efforts to solve some of the problems of rural health care. In 1946, the U.S. Congress passed the Hill-Burton Act, which provided federal subsidy to states and communities for hospital development. Many of the hospitals constructed in small towns and cities throughout the United States since World War II owe their existence to funds derived from this legislation. The belief that a small hospital would serve as a focus for health care for parts of rural America, however, is unfounded. Many of these hospitals are struggling to stay open. The sophistication of modern hospital care requires staffing with personnel not always available in small towns. The expense of maintaining hospitals is often too much for the poor rural areas they serve. Again, the need to care for inpatients creates another burden for the busy medical practitioner. Whatever the reasons, the hospitals developed in rural areas as a result of the Hill-Burton legislation have not reversed the trend of decreasing health services. Although good hospital facilities do attract and encourage young physicians to establish nearby practices, this has not been true in small rural towns.

The Sears Roebuck Foundation began in 1957 to work with rural regions to help them recruit physicians. The foundation provided the community with the expertise to decide whether it had the economic base to support one physician or more. If the results were satisfactory, the foundation and the community would construct a professional office building. Conceivably, this would lure the young physician to set up a medical practice. At first, many doctors were impressed by these visible indicators of a community's desire to have them and particularly its desire to minimize the economic impediments to starting practice. Unfortunately, this effort by the Sears Roebuck Foundation has not been successful. At least half of these buildings stand empty. Doctors come with good intentions, and after a few years leave for some of the reasons already stated. The foundation is no longer directing its efforts to help rural communities recruit doctors.

Recently, the federal government, through the U.S. Public Health Service, has been trying to encourage health professionals of all types to locate in communities badly needing their services. This includes the densely impacted urban areas as well as the rural villages. In an admittedly trial venture, Congress has provided funds to establish a National Health Service Corps, composed of young health professionals who have become commissioned officers of the U.S. Public Health Service. Again, communities must apply to the Public Health Service, indicating their willingness to participate and defining their need for medical services. Initially, the local and state medical societies were asked to agree to the need of the community for medical and other health services; this stipulation has recently been revoked. If the application of the community is favorably reviewed, it may then be assigned a doctor and / or dentist or other health professional. Together the community and the Public Health Service arrange the place for practice and purchase the necessary equipment. For two years, the physician may remain a commissioned officer and be paid by the government. His fees go to a community board which has the option of spending them for improving health services or returning them to the federal treasury.

At this time, less than two hundred physicians have been assigned in this fashion, the majority to rural communities. It is too early to tell how many will stay and serve in the community. It is difficult to assess the abolition of the doctor's draft law and its impact on the recruitment of young physicians into the National Health Service Corps. Unfortunately, while this project appeals to the altruism of enthusiastic young health professionals, it does not solve the chronic problems of recruiting and maintaining health professionals in rural communities whose basic social structure is at odds with the attitudes of the professionals and their families. With the conclusion of the military involvement in Southeast Asia, and the discontinuation of the doctor's draft law, it remains to be seen how many doctors will opt for such a career choice. Fortunately, the two hundred or so health professionals who have been assigned at this time (August 1973) should indicate in two years the degree of success or failure of this program.

Even this brief outline of problems involved in changing patterns of rural health care suggests that there are no simple solutions. The belief that training more physicians in the hope that increased numbers will result in a spillover of leftover medical talent into rural America is not well founded. Similarly, the education of more physicians in general or family medicine has little to do with the choice of practice setting. What, then, might work to improve health care services for rural populations?

Any system of health care planned for rural areas must have concern for the needs and expectations both of the rural citizens and of the health professionals. This system will have to involve many different health professionals working in concert to deliver health care to a sparse population. The key to rural health care is in the development of a system. Individual entrepreneurship of a solo general practitioner will not work.

Chapter III in this book describes the content of rural health care. This analysis suggests that many illnesses seen in a primary health care clinic can be adequately handled by a physician's assistant or a nurse practitioner working with a physician. In a nearby doctorless county, this same Department of Community Health and Family Medicine which sponsored the Lafayette County Health Center has developed a primary health care clinic staffed by two physician's assistants (PAs), a licensed practical nurse (LPN), and a clerk-receptionist. Doctors visit the clinic daily to review the records of each patient encountered and consult with the physician's assistant. The organization and performance of this clinic has been described. Suffice it to say that this rural community does accept PAs as purveyors of health care. The faculty supervisors are convinced that good quality health care is practiced. Ample investigative work has been done by others to conclude that excellent health care is provided by nurse practitioners or physicians; this includes the pediatric nurse practitioners trained by Dr. Silver in Denver and the nurse practitioner program of Dr. Lewis in Kansas. The conclusion is that someone other than a physician is able to provide primary health care. But this individual needs to be answerable to and under the supervision of a physician or group of physicians. This supervision does not require immediate proximity but can result from scheduled visits, telephone conversations, and perhaps in the future closed circuit television.

It is plausible, then, to conceive of a network of care serving a defined rural area. Primary care would be provided by physician's assistants or nurse practitioners. This would be monitored by physicians through some mechanism insuring quality of care but not necessarily requiring the immediate presence of a physician. Physicians would be responsible for developing preventive medicine programs directed in part at school health, appropriate immunizations, cancer screening, and diabetes and hypertension detection. Maintenance care for individuals with chronic illness would result from a partnership of effort between the paramedical assistant and the physician. Provision for recognition and treatment of mental illness can utilize a similar effort. The involvement of the patient in his own health care is important. This effective partnership between patient and health professional can result from consumer health education including programs interspersed in elementary and high schools. Physicians would be available for most secondary and all tertiary care.

Under this scheme of an umbrella of health care for a defined rural region, small groups of physicians, preferably those trained in family medicine, would work as a unit, with paramedical professionals assuming the responsibility for the health of a community. They would employ and, where necessary, train the appropriate health assistants to accomplish this mission. In turn, the family physicians would consult with other doctors with specialty skills necessary to treat the esoteric or unusual illness. The content of community medical practice requires only the availability of those specialized talents, which would most likely be present in a large city with an appropriate hospital for sophisticated care, the service region of which would include the rural area. The economics and organization of such a system could develop between a combination of national health insurance and a health maintenance organization.

There are impediments to such a proposed network of health

care. Included in this chapter are allusions to the expectations of community members for health care. They would have to change their allegiance from a person responsible for health care to a system or organization and accept a significant amount of their care from someone other than a physician. Hopefully through health education programs, patients would become major participants in their own health care. This scheme of health care stresses prevention of illness and maintenance of health as well as the treatment of episodic illness. Physicians, to function in this system, need consequently to relinquish some of the intimacy of their patient relationships. It requires the recognition and acceptance that many physician's tasks can be performed satisfactorily by someone with lesser training. In rural regions, only one such network of care would be available. Competing organizations of health care delivery probably could not survive in sparsely populated regions. This creates the problem that dissatisfied constituents would conceivably have to leave the region to seek health care.

Some innovation and imagination is necessary to address the immediate problem of rural health care. That present methods of organized health care have deteriorated or almost disappeared in many rural regions may ease the restraints to change. Whatever the proposed changes are, however, the social structures and patterns of the rural residents concerning health care and their expectations for health care must be recognized and understood. The professionals—doctors, nurses, physicians' assistants—will need to undergo similar changes in their concepts of health care. The need for experiments in rural health care delivery is obvious. Presently they can be undertaken only with subsidy of grants from government or foundations. Perhaps with enactment of national health insurance, groups of physicians or selected medical schools would find it economically possible to undertake major projects in rural health care.

V. The Doctor in the Rural County

Richard A. Henry, M.D.

A FUNDAMENTAL DIMENSION of health care in the rural community concerns the practicing physician and his experiences. As an introductory framework for the material of this chapter, therefore, one rural practitioner of fifteen years' standing was asked to recall a typical day in his practice.

A recitation of typical activities of the rural solo general practitioner will do little for the physician who has been there, but for other readers it may provide some insight.

The usual and routine day, first of all, does not exist. If there is a constancy about any day, it is that it is busy, filled with what might seem to be repetitive problems but, considering the kaleidoscope of each individual's genes, circumstances, attitudes and beliefs, family, work, education, and experience, it is, in reality, unending variation. The stuffy nose is not a stuffy nose standing alone. It is housed in a body subject to all the influences enumerated above. It isn't just a discomfort; it is embarrassing, it interferes with work or plans, it means "something else" is going on, the rest of the family can catch it, and there is some measure of expectation of reassurance and / or relief.

Hospital rounds are first on the agenda. If the schedule is not preempted by an emergency call for the patients who "toughed it out" through the night but couldn't last after 6:00 A.M., they begin at 7:00 A.M. Ten patients are seen, progress notes written, an admission note is written for the patient to be admitted later—then, to the operating room.

One of the more peaceful parts of the day occurs in surgery. In assisting at surgery, or in performing that surgery in which one is competent, there is a serenity which comes from the aura of regimentation and ritual. Everyone knows his function, and even the unexpected has limitations on its variability. The difficult bleeder, the cardiac arrest, and the technical challenges have been anticipated and the shift in activity to correct them is smooth and almost automatic. Should the procedure last three to four hours, it is strange that the tired legs and aching back are noticeable only when the dressing is being applied.

A few more tasks which have accumulated during surgery require attention at the hospital, and then the office hours begin. Once in the office, there is a brief time for a good-morning chat and coffee with the staff. Office practice is usually a blur of unrelenting activity lasting until 5:30 or 6:00 P.M.—first one room, then another, and back to the first, to the lab, to the x-ray room, and to the office to look up something. You schedule thirty patients when forty want appointments that day, knowing full well that you will have ten drop-ins whom you cannot refuse for one reason or another, plus one or two lacerations, splinters, or a patient with a foreign body in his eye. In each room there is a patient with a different problem or set of problems, or different conditions to be met in addressing a similar problem.

The telephone calls from out of town and the emergency calls are answered. The routine calls are stacked on the desk to be answered during the two or three periods set aside for them during the day, while the feet rest on the desk. Lunch is a brown paper bag in the coffee room. It seems a shame to have patients waiting in the office while you drive home for a comfortable lunch.

Home calls, I feel, are a reasonable and humanistic part of any practice; furthermore, provided the physician limits the number to those for whom he determines it is indicated (i.e., the patients whose health will be *better* served by seeing them at home), the experience can be rewarding and educational with regard to the circumstances in which the patient lives. In my practice, I averaged two to three house calls each day and found them well worthwhile. They are worked into the day's schedule whenever possible.

In the evening there is a return to the hospital for rounds and to complete the work-ups on any new admissions. When on call for the emergency room, this may be the fifth visit to the hospital that day; on those days when one tries to get out of the office promptly at 5:00 P.M.there are likely to be twenty to thirty more patients that evening in the emergency room. Needless to say, you do not make any other plans for those days.

When not on call, the feeling upon leaving the hospital or the last house call for the day is one of pleasant exhilaration. There is a genuine excitement about having a choice, which you feel you have well earned, about which way you will drive home, and what drink or appetizer you will have with your relaxed conversation or silence with your wife. Of course, there are a few more telephone calls during the evening, some requiring you to go out again; no one, however, expects you to do anything but temporize (except in true emergencies), so you feel fairly confident that the interruption will be brief.

Frankly, there's not much left in you at the end of a "usual" day for avocations or hobbies. You can be quite content with a variety of activities, none of which are considered seriously, because you know the next day will require all the energy and enthusiasm you can produce.

And what does all this get you? Aside from the problems of maintaining some kind of balance for your family life, obtaining your continuing education and needed exercise and recreation, the practice of medicine provides more interest, challenge, and greater rewards per minute than any other activity I know. Four years after leaving practice, I asked some of my former patients who are farmers whether they could plant a field in a special type of grass I wanted for haying. (Of course, I acquired a small farm during my practice.) On the appointed day they showed up with several huge tractors, assorted equipment, and a small army of men who knew what they were doing. They planted my 40-acre hay field in six hours, even with my inept assistance. After it was all over, I asked them what I could pay (expecting a cost of at least $2,000). They replied that I could not pay them anything for their work or their machines. Not only that , but the workers would not take any money either. Where today can you find such a concrete expression of friendship as that?

Rural citizens identify their family physician as the most desirable provider of personal health care. They want a doctor with whom they feel comfortable, in whom they can confide, and who is readily available. On the other hand, doctors in rural communities often feel that their patients want to own and possess, love and idealize them all at the same time.

Rural medical practice is rigorous. The patient demands are great. The hours of work are long. Individual and family privacy is virtually impossible. In the rural area little anonymity exists for the physician. In time all idiosyncrasies and habits become well known. This is equally true for the family of the physician. The doctor must realize that his personal and professional mishaps will become known to the community. He will also realize that rural citizens are often more tolerant of human error. Until recently malpractice suits against rural physicians were uncommon.

Professional isolation does occur to those physicians who do not have the self-discipline necessary to structure their practice and postgraduate education in such a way as to provide continuous communication and consultation with their peers. The larger medical community (the state and county medical societies, various professional organizations) responds to the need for continuing education by sponsoring numerous programs enabling the interested physician to keep up. The doctor who takes half a day a week from his practice for graduate educational activities hurts neither his practice nor his patients. This activity is essential for the rural physician, if he is to remain dynamic in his approach to medical practice. Understandably, there is always difficulty in the face of immediate patient demands in taking time out for continuing education.

The established rural physician is usually near the top of the prestige pyramid. This may result in ascribing to him authority in areas completely outside his field of knowledge, and in endowing him with the ability to address problems in religion, finance, and world affairs.

It is important for the rural physician to discipline himself against assuming these areas of expertise. Apportioning some sacrosanct time each week for activities totally unrelated to medicine is perhaps the best way to regain needed perspective and to remember his feet of clay.

Rewards of rural practice for physicians include, however, a sense of belonging and need in a community, long-term intimate patient relationships, and a significant visible contribution to the health of many people.

Inevitably, in rural practice, one develops an intimate rapport with an enlarging, dependent family of patients. The stable residence of many rural families enhances this physician-patient closeness. The physician knows the members of a family, their political and religious attitudes, their economic status, educational levels, their aspirations for the future. He shares with them in a very personal way their triumphs and disappointments.

Rural communities provide a suitable environment for rearing children. Stable, long-standing friendships are possible for children. Delinquency is uncommon. To grow up in a small town, to work part-time at different jobs while in school, are cherishable opportunities for children offered in many rural settings.

For the physician and his family, there is ample and varied social life in any rural community. In fact, the temptation, frequently, is that there are too many social opportunities. The physician needs judgment in order to apportion his time wisely. Local government, civic clubs, the hunters' club, the football weekenders' club, the chamber of commerce, the church, all of these will claim some of the physician's time. To participate in these activities will permit the physician to know better his community and its citizens. He must be selective in his participation, however, or his limited time for these ventures will be spread too thin and he will be ineffective.

In many rural areas recreational opportunities are magnificent. Hunting and fishing, hiking and camping facilities are usually nearby. Golf courses and tennis courts are not crowded. One can travel to the nearby town for different entertainment and then leave its congestion and traffic problems behind. For the rural doctor the hitch is in trying to find the time to participate in these opportunities.

Adequate remuneration in a rural general practice is the least of the physician's worries. It is necessary that he recognize the fact that he is running a business which includes consideration of salaries, insurance, capital, rent, and depreciation. Once recognized, the efficient physician delegates these responsibilities to experts in these fields (except for policy decisions) and proceeds to practice medicine. When I started my practice, my main concern was whether there would be enough income to meet my needs and expectations. A friend told me that, after the first year, my main concern would be having enough to pay income taxes. He was right.

If the life of a rural physician is rewarding, productive, and remunerative and the rural setting is a pleasant place to live and raise a family, why are the numbers of rural physicians dwindling? All health manpower reports clearly show that few doctors are entering rural areas to practice. Until recently fewer doctors were being trained as family physicians with the appropriate skills of medicine and surgery particularly suited to rural practice. The obvious conclusion is that there are decreasing numbers of doctors to serve rural residents, and the average age of those who are practicing in rural areas is slowly increasing. As the older physicians die or retire, another rural community is left without the services of a doctor.

Little is known of the practice and work habits of the rural physician in this country. For the most part he is too busy to scrutinize his own practice and often too far from academic health centers to be included in their perusal.

Recently (1973), Dr. Frank Sloan and his associates in the Department of Economics of the University of Florida surveyed thirty-two randomly selected family physicians from among a family practitioner population of 274 in north central Florida. For purposes of the study, the group was subdivided into physicians under and over age fifty and into those who practiced in metropolitan and non-metropolitan communities. In north central Florida a physician working in a nonmetropolitan community is engaged in a rural practice.

The statistics he has gathered are rather penetrating in revealing the fallacy of physician-population ratios as a guide to availability of health care. Governmental agencies and medical organizations traditionally have used this ratio as a yardstick of accessibility; without the qualifications depicted in this study, however, such ratios are obviously deceptive.

Table 1 contains some professional characteristics of the younger and the mature family physician according to his site of practice. Twenty-five percent of the general physicians under age fifty no longer accept new patients compared to one-half of that percentage for doctors over age fifty. Obstetrics is not practiced by three-fourths of these physicians.

It takes nearly two to three weeks to schedule an appointment with a physician for a physical examination; for a nonacute medical problem, the wait for appointment varies between one and two weeks. Approximately 5 percent of the patients seen by this group of general practitioners are referred to other doctors. None of the groups of doctors in this survey averaged more than two housecalls a week.

Younger physicians tended to schedule more patients than the older generalists. One-quarter of the latter in rural communities still operate on a first-come–first-served basis. Metropolitan physicians appeared to be more rigid in their scheduling of patient visits, with

TABLE 1

PHYSICIAN AVAILABILITY CHARACTERISTICS

	Nonmetropolitan		Metropolitan	
	Under 50	50 and +	Under 50	50 and +
Access				
% accepting *no* new patients	25.0	12.5	25.0	12.5
% accepting all patients	12.5	12.5	0.0	12.5
Scheduling				
Delay in receiving appointment				
(days)—for physical exam	23.6	13.3	21.9	18.5
for nonacute illness	15.8	6.0	6.5	7.9
for acute illness	1.0	0.38	1.13	0.88
% of patient visits scheduled	71.9	32.4	77.3	88.0
% of MDs who do *no* scheduling	12.5	25.0	0.0	0.0
% of MDs who do *not* have open				
clinic hours	62.5	37.5	87.5	75.0
Patient Waiting Time in Office				
If patient has scheduled app't.	34.5	13.1	15.3	39.1
During MDs' open clinic hours*	13.1	18.1	9.4	26.3
If patient arrives without app't.				
when MD is seeing scheduled				
patients ("drop-in")	112.9	50.6	42.9	52.5
Referrals and Telephone				
% of patient visits ending in				
referrals to other MDs	5.5	6.0	6.1	4.9
Telephone calls per MD (day)				
for consultations that do not				
result in visit	7.5	7.9	10.3	9.8
Telephone calls for entire practice				
(day) for consultations that do				
not result in visit	23.4	17.6	16.5	22.0
Visit Mix				
Home visits per week	2.0	1.6	1.3	1.0
% MDs who do not make home calls	50.0	50.0	50.0	75.0
% who do not accept pediatric p'ts.	0.0	12.5	12.5	37.5
% who do not perform maternity				
services	62.5	75.0	75.0	75.0
Hours of Work				
Total hours per week	55.8	44.8	47.0	44.8
Direct p't. care hrs. per week	49.1	41.1	41.5	40.8
Office hours per week	29.6	30.5	30.1	26.1
Direct p't. care hrs. / 100 hrs.	0.89	0.92	0.89	0.93
Length of Visit (minutes)				
Physical exam—scheduled time	40.6	31.4	46.3	28.1
MD time	27.3	20.4	30.0	23.5
Nonacute illness—scheduled time	14.4	13.4	15.0	11.3
MD time	9.1	11.0	11.6	9.0
Acute illness—scheduled time	13.8	15.3	13.1	15.6
MD time	8.4	12.5	10.0	11.5

* Hours set aside for seeing patients on a nonscheduled basis.

only a few maintaining open clinic hours set aside each day for seeing patients on a nonscheduled basis.

The total hours of work per week for a rural general practitioner under age fifty are nearly fifty-six. This is deceptive, however, as it depicts only those hours actually worked. These doctors are available many hours that they are not working. This availability precludes their participation in many activities enjoyed by others.

Table 2 contains some other practice characteristics of these same general physicians. The rural physician under age fifty has by far the most patient contact, averaging nearly 300 per week. Of these,

TABLE 2

OTHER PRACTICE CHARACTERISTICS

| | Nonmetropolitan | | Metropolitan | |
	Under 50	50 and +	Under 50	50 and +
Visits (per week)				
Total visits	299	235	176	209
Office visits	196	176	140	159
Hospital visits	94	49	32	39
Aides per MD	4.6	3.7	3.4	2.6

196 are seen in the office, 94 are visited in the hospital, and the remaining few at home, in nursing homes, or in the emergency room of the local hospital. Because of this patient work load, these rural practitioners employ on the average of 4.6 persons in their offices.

Why then would a physician choose a rural community in which to practice, and stay, as so many of them do, for the duration of their professional lives? The reasons are as varied as the individuals themselves. The largest single determining factor for locating in a rural community is the rural heritage of the physician and his spouse. But this accounts for less than half of the rural physician population.

Most medical education occurs in the metropolitan areas, and doctors settle near the communities in which they train. Current medical education emphasizes specialty training and the need for sophisticated supportive services, particularly in x-ray and laboratory diagnoses. There is also a tendency for young doctors to practice in groups, which permit them to share the expenses of practice and the problems of being on call on nights and weekends. In group practices, time is more easily arranged for vacations and postgraduate education.

Rural physicians have characteristically been solo general practitioners. It is doubtful whether the present genesis of family practice residency programs will result in an increase in the number of rural doctors unless they train their residents to work in teams of physicians and new health care assistants and adapt to a rural practice.

In the chapter "The Content of Rural Medical Practice," the concept that many of the ills for which patients seek medical care are minor and self-limiting is supported. These health and medical needs could be met by someone other than a physician. Conceivably a nurse-practitioner or a physician's assistant working under the supervision of a physician would be able to assume responsibility for providing many of these services.

The experiences of the medical school faculty, residents, and students while providing health care to the residents of Lafayette County confirmed the impression that someone other than a physician would be able to respond to most of the health needs of a rural population. An experiment in rural health care was then designed to test the hypothesis, that physician's assistants would perform satisfactorily while geographically separate from but still responsible to physicians. An attempt was made to answer these questions:

1. Would the community accept the physician's assistant as a provider of ambulatory health care?

2. Would the physician's assistants be personally satisfied with the rewards of practice and their role in the community?

3. Would the quality of care be good enough to satisfy the medical school faculty?

The physician's assistant is able to perform adequately and completely the routine repetitive tasks that physicians traditionally do, and he is competent to assess the needs of patients in primary health care. Specific tasks he may accomplish are:

Prenatal examination	Premarital examination
Newborn examination	Preemployment examination
Preschool examination	Insurance examination

Initial patient evaluation of a specific complaint

Complete routine examination
Monitoring of chronic diseases such as arthritis, diabetes, and
    hypertension
Advice on diets and regimens
Treatment of minor lacerations and bruises
Examination and treatment of common self-limiting illnesses

The list in itself is impressive. Even more impressive is the amount of time spent every day on these tasks by the physician.

The study began in August 1971 in Trenton (Gilchrist County), Florida, 30 miles west of Gainesville. The county population is 3,500. This county was selected because of its geographic proximity to the College of Medicine and also because it represented similar rural counties in Florida where there are no or few physicians. This county had been without a physician for five years. There are four such counties in Florida and 134 counties in the United States that are similarly situated. Most of these are agriculturally dependent communities which are thinly populated.

Through the cooperation of the Gilchrist County Commissioners and interested members of the community, a clinic was established employing two physician's assistants who were directed and supervised by faculty from the University of Florida College of Medicine. Prior approval for this project was obtained from the Florida Medical Association as well as from the Medical Advisory Committee to the University of Florida College of Medicine.

Two and one-half months after the clinic opened, 100 consecutive patients were contacted by mail, two weeks after their visit to the clinic. The survey was directed at determining the patients' subjective acceptance of health services provided by the physician's assistants. Patients were also asked how they planned to use the clinic for health services in the future. Would they limit themselves only to emergency medical services and minor illness needs, or would the clinic be the point of entry for all health care?

Sixty-five of these questionnaires were returned and the nonrespondents were followed up by home visits. There were no differences in the replies of those who sent back the questionnaires and those interviewed at home. Ninty-five percent of the patients perceived the service as competent, thorough, efficacious, and courteous. Five percent thought it was not. One complaint was that the wait to see the physician's assistant was too long; another was a misunderstanding about fees. There were no complaints regarding quality of service. Eighty-five percent of the residents stated that they would use the clinic for all of their health care problems and 15 percent stated that they would use it for minor injuries and illnesses and go elsewhere for major problems.

Clinic attendance has grown steadily since the beginning of activities. Two years later, twenty-five patients a day are seen at the clinic. Acceptance of working and living in the rural county by the physician's assistants has been good. One physician's assistant left because of a personal family problem but volunteered that he thoroughly enjoyed his work and role in the clinic. He has since been replaced by another physician's assistant.

Acceptance of the actual work of the physician's assistant by those physicians who have traditionally treated these patients has been difficult to measure. Sixteen physicians in the surrounding communities were identified as usually treating the majority of patients in the county. Presently an increasing number of these physicians are suggesting to their patients that they get a test done or blood pressure taken, or get their cast looked at or their sutures removed, by the physician's assistant in the community. Perhaps this reflects some acceptance by these practicing physicians.

Most difficult to determine is the quality of health care delivered by the physician's assistant. Each patient encounter is recorded by the physician's assistant on a stylized problem-oriented medical record. Each day a physician from the Department of Community Health and Family Medicine visits the clinic and reviews these records. In addition, the physician is available for consultation with patients or discussions of medical topics or patient problems with the physician's assistant. Subjectively the physicians who monitor the medical services of the physician's assistants are convinced that they do a highly acceptable job. This conclusion is the result of reviewing the medical records, talking with the physician's assistants, and seeing patients in consultation with them. Probably no other primary care practice has such scrutiny as the physician's assistants working in Gilchrist County.

Present indications are that 80 percent of the patients seen at the clinic are taken care of competently by the physician's assistants without any physician input. In the case of 10 percent of the patients, the physician's assistants like to discuss the patient with a physician but do not need a formal consultation. Ten percent of the patients reviewed by the physician's assistants require a consultation with a physician.

A more sophisticated study is underway, using computer analysis of patient records as a possible mechanism of gauging the quality of medical practice. For example, this study will enable the reviewer to determine what percentage of upper respiratory infections in various age groups is treated with antibiotics. Plans are also being developed to explore the possible use of closed circuit television interviews as an adjunct to supervising the activities of the physician's assistants.

Despite the advantages of practicing in rural communities, some of which have been noted in this chapter, doctors will return to rural practice settings only if new concepts of medical practice are introduced. Probably the two greatest changes in practice now underway are the sharing of the problems and rigors of practice by groups of physicians and the delegation of a significant portion of the responsibility for medical services to paramedical personnel; the intensive and coronary care nurses are one example of the latter.

The physician's assistant is not the final answer to personal, primary medical services for rural residents. The utilization of physician's assistants in rural settings as part of a system of health care, however, may represent a feasible response to some of the health care needs of rural citizens.

The rural community must alter its expectation of health care. Trying to attract solo general practitioners to continue the health care style of yesteryear has not worked for several decades. The rural community needs to understand the wisdom of receiving its medical services from groups of doctors and paramedical personnel. Most important, the rural citizenry should work with health professionals in defining their health care needs and both groups should respond by evolving the best system of health care for a specific community.

Studies in Rural Health

THE CHAPTERS IN THIS SECTION share a common theme: the interrelationship between Lafayette County residents' attitudes toward health and care, their perceived level of functioning, their use of health facilities, and their actual state of well-being.

The first study explores the health care attitudes of culturally disadvantaged rural residents, delineating a cluster of expectations and behavioral characteristics toward health. The effect of deprivation upon the patient's attitudes toward self is considered, and suggestions are made for the incorporation of these findings into health planning.

The second study describes the unusually high incidence of emotional impairment in this rural county, relating the findings to family income, education, age, and racial characteristics of the population. There is discussion of the effect of psychosocial impairment on the patient's health-seeking behavior, loss of functional effectiveness, family mental and physical illness patterns, and perception of one's own general health.

The studies of folk remedies in Lafayette County describe the strong effect of folk beliefs on health practices in a contemporary rural community. The development and characteristics of folk beliefs are discussed, and the author offers a careful examination of these beliefs surrounding one modern clinical procedure, the "shot" or injection.

The final chapter in this section reports a unique study of the communication patterns between black patients and physicians at the rural health center. Data from medical records are compared with patient interview responses to determine the degree of agreement and consensus in these communications concerning the patient's health and care. Suggestions are made for improving communication patterns.

VI. The Meaning of Deprivation
Health Care Attitudes of Disadvantaged Rural Groups

Sam A. Banks, Ph.D.

RESEARCHERS ENGAGED IN THE STUDY of health attitudes must resist two prevalent but unacknowledged fallacies. The first is a portrayal of the subject population as a collection of passive objects with stable characteristics that can easily be measured (if they will only hold still long enough!). This oversimplification reduces the complexity of the task and the anxiety of the researcher, but it does not do justice to the richness and creativity of the persons studied. It is equally dangerous to view the researcher as a value-sanitized, empty receptacle into which interview data are poured. Any study of health attitudes is an active dialogue, shaped by both the studier and the studied. This inquiry regarding health care attitudes resulted from the interplay between the University of Florida Department of Community Health faculty's concerns (embedded in the research design) and Lafayette County residents' needs (expressed in the information derived).

During the course of projects such as the one described in this chapter, "target populations" have a disturbing and creative tendency to become co-researchers. The persons interviewed have issues to pose. Questions long muffled by the routine of community life are amplified under the stimulus of the interview setting. The foundations for such consumer participation had been unusually well laid in

Lafayette County. For three years prior to the study, physicians from the Department of Community Health and Family Medicine had been offering comprehensive health care to the residents of Lafayette County through a clinic located in Mayo, the county seat. The exploration of these residents' views regarding their health and care was a natural consequence of this ongoing interchange.

During the design and analysis of the interviews, three questions emerged as significant foci for the researchers and the residents. The first dealt with the relationship between the forms of disability, emotional and physical, experienced by people in the county. In Chapter VII, Dr. George Warheit has examined the incidence of emotional impairment among the Lafayette County population and the correlation between degree of impairment and specific health attitudes.

The second group of findings compared clinic patient families with those not utilizing this facility. While the information will not be treated in detail in this chapter, some findings are of interest. The subpopulation of clinic users numbered a significantly larger proportion of the young, the black, the poor, and those with less education. When compared with the nonclinic county population, these patients saw their physicians as respecting them, caring for them, listening to them, understanding them, and taking more time with them than did the other group.

The third portion of the study, comprising the remainder of this chapter, highlights the effect of deprivation on the health-related attitudes of these rural citizens. There has been a continual outflow of "the best and the brightest" from rural areas to the city. The remaining precipitate offers a chance to study the magnified effects of aging, poverty, lack of educational opportunity, and racial repression on human beings' responses to health care.

SIGNIFICANCE

Increased national concern and expenditure for health care underlines the necessity for greater understanding of Americans' attitudes regarding the state of their health and the forms of care that they find acceptable. In 1970, our country spent over $67 billion for health care. This concern for the enhancement of citizens' physical and emotional well-being is matched by a growing awareness that health care planning should take into account measures to provide financial security, educational opportunity, satisfactory living conditions for the aging, and racial equality. If these problems are interlinked (and their solutions interdependent), it is important to consider the nature of that relationship.

Further, the large size of our poor, black, undereducated, or aging populations demands that they receive a hearing. In 1970, 12.6 percent of all noninstitutionalized Americans had a family income below the poverty line. One of every four citizens over twenty-five years old had not received any high school education. One in five persons in the United States was over fifty-five years old. There were 22,580,000 black Americans, an increase of 20 percent over the 1960 total. Public concern for these groups is reflected in federal and state budgets. Governmentally funded health care for the aging cost over $7 billion in 1970.

The following paragraphs, focusing on the health care attitudes of these disadvantaged groups in rural areas, draw upon findings of a study of Lafayette County residents' views regarding their health and their expectations about health care.

RESEARCH DESIGN

From May 1970 to June 1971, members of the Department of Community Health and Family Medicine, University of Florida College of Medicine, studied the health care attitudes of residents in a north Florida rural county (Lafayette). The project was conducted under a grant provided by the Bureau of Comprehensive Health Planning, Florida State Board of Health. Two graduate students in the health sciences, specifically trained and supervised for the purpose, interviewed a stratified random sample of 126 adults in their homes. The interviews contained 80 items designed to yield both free descriptive responses and structured statistical data. Interviews averaged one and one-half hours in length.

Findings of the study include appropriate demographic data, interviewees' self-assessments of past and present health, and their current attitudes and ideal expectations concerning the state and care of their health in the following areas:

1. Symptoms and conditions requiring care
2. Length of time elapsing between recognition of illness and request for health care

3. Settings in which and personnel from whom health care is received and desired
4. Characteristics of the relationship with health professionals experienced and desired by the patient
5. Results received and expected from health care
6. Payment transactions adopted and desired
7. Perceived barriers or impediments to desired care

The major independent variables considered and compared in analyzing the data were race, age, sex, level of education, family income, and psychological impairment scores (Leighton Health Opinion Survey). Two primary statistical measures were used: frequency histograms (to describe the overall population sample) and Pearson's chi square statistic (for comparison and contrast of subgroups).

GENERAL FINDINGS

The study sample reveals a people embedded in a rural life style. Fifty-six percent grew up on farms or in towns of less than 2,500. The population is unusually stable. While a significant number of the young move to urban areas, 44.4 percent of the sample had always lived in Lafayette County, 76.1 percent in northern Florida.

It is interesting to note the heavy proportion of the aging, undereducated, poor, and emotionally impaired among the residents of the county. Thirty-seven percent of the respondents were over sixty years of age; only 19 percent of the United States population were over fifty-five in 1970. Similarly, 71.3 percent of the rural sample were older than forty years, while only 41.8 percent of the 1970 United States population were over thirty-five. Study findings reveal a distinctly low educational level. While only 27.8 percent of Americans over twenty-five years of age have less than a high school education, 44 percent of the rural Florida sample have not attended high school.

The prevalence of poverty is marked. Only 14 percent of the families in the United States had incomes under $4,000 in 1970. In contrast, 60 percent of the Lafayette County sample reported equally low incomes. Approximately one-half of the families in the United States reported annual incomes of less than $10,000. It is striking that over three-fourths of the rural county families had incomes under $8,000. When one considers that 31 percent of the families studied had more than one wage earner (and that 11.9 percent of the people had more than one job), this low level of family income is indicative of underpayment rather than underemployment. More people in a poor rural family must work at more jobs in order to subsist.

The degree of emotional impairment within the sample was evaluated through responses to the Leighton Health Opinion Survey items. The validity of this scale has been confirmed in recent comparisons with forty-three other measures in the Southern Mental Health Needs and Services Study, conducted by John J. Schwab, M.D. and George J. Warheit, Ph.D. The scale results indicate that 23.8 percent of the Lafayette County sample suffer serious emotional impairment and that 49.2 percent are at least moderately impaired. It is interesting that the mean level of impairment in the overall sample is the same as that found in a group of selected emotionally disturbed patients from a nearby semiurban county (Alachua County). The general populations tested in Alachua County indicated only 7 percent seriously and 25 percent moderately impaired. It is estimated that 20 percent of adult Americans suffer moderate impairment.

COMPARATIVE FINDINGS

In comparing population subgroups according to race, age, sex, education, family income, and psychological impairment scores, distinct clusters of attitudes held in common by these groups emerged, with one exception. No statistically significant attitudinal differences were obtained between men and women. It should be noted, however, that blackness, low individual and family income, and low educational level were significantly related. Similarly, aging groups were significantly less educated, less employed, and had lower individual and family incomes. The undereducated group contained more blacks, elderly, unemployed, low income, and emotionally impaired people. The low income group had significantly more black, aging, undereducated, unemployed, and emotionally impaired individuals (Table 1).

Blacks were not more significantly emotionally impaired than whites, nor did the aging reveal more emotional dysfunction than younger groups. There was evidence, however, of greater impairment among the undereducated and the poor (Table 1).

As these rural groups view their past and present health, they consistently report a lower level of functioning and of experienced

TABLE 1

RELATIONSHIPS AMONG DISADVANTAGED GROUPS IN RURAL SAMPLE

	Blacks More Than Whites	Aging More Than Younger	Lower Education More Than Higher Education	Lower Family Income More Than Higher Family Income	Seriously Emotionally Impaired More Than Minimally Impaired
More blacks	—	N.S.	p<.001	p<.001	N.S.
More aging members	N.S.	—	p<.001	p<.001	N.S.
More undereducated members	p<.001	p<.001	—	p<.001	p<.05
More low family income members	p<.001	p<.001	p<.001	—	p<.05
More emotionally impaired members	N.S.	N.S.	p<.05	p<.05	—

(N.S. = Not Significant)

well-being. All five subpopulations report significantly poorer general health. All feel distinctly less "healthy enough to carry out the things I would like to do." Aging and emotionally impaired groups state significantly more often than the younger and less impaired that they "have to go easy on work because of poor health." When compared with others, lower education and income groups and those more severely impaired indicate a greater frequency of "periods of days, weeks, or months, when I can't get going." The elderly, undereducated, and emotionally impaired report a distinct worsening of their health during the last five years (as compared to younger, more educated, and less impaired individuals). Those with less education and those with poor emotional health (as reflected by the Leighton Survey) report more often that their work affects their health adversely (Table 2).

Previous studies have indicated a "high incidence of remediable conditions together with low rates of utilization for the poor, the black, and the other socially disadvantaged population groups." The attitudes reflected by these groups in the sample shed some light on the causes for their low utilization of health resources. The disadvantaged tend to seek a narrow range of care, defining only acute and serious illnesses and trauma as deserving treatment; the less educated seek and want less preventive care (p<.05), desire fewer check-ups (p<.05). Such health aids as glasses are far less important to the undereducated (p<.01). The poor indicate the same attitude toward check-ups (p<.05) and health aids (p<.05). These attitudes do not reflect less *need* for health care on the part of the disadvantaged. On the contrary, Louis Harris has reported a significantly higher incidence of medical problems among these patients.

On experiencing illness, the disadvantaged rural patients in our sample delayed their search for professional care significantly longer than other groups. The poor (p<.01) and blacks (p<.05) report that they "wait until I just can't go on" much more than whites and the more affluent. They indicate that, if health care could be just as they wish, they would still wait until they "cannot go on" (p<.01). Blacks and the poor use the dentist less (p<.05). Both groups use physicians less (p<.01), and blacks would *expect* to use one less, even under ideal conditions (p<.05). On the other hand, these groups and the less educated turn to religious healers, "persons with powers," and supernatural aid more often than do whites and those with more income (p<.001).

TABLE 2

SELF-REPORTS OF PAST AND PRESENT HEALTH BY DISADVANTAGED GROUPS

	Blacks More Than Whites	Aging More Than Younger	Lower Education More Than Higher Education	Lower Family Income More Than Higher Family Income	Seriously Emotionally Impaired More Than Minimally Impaired
Report general health poorer	$p<.02$	$p<.01$	$p<.001$	$p<.01$	$p<.001$
Have periods where can't get going	N.S.	N.S.	$p<.01$	$p<.01$	$p<.001$
Have had to go easy on work because of poor health	N.S.	$p<.01$	N.S.	N.S.	$p<.001$
Don't feel healthy enough to carry out what would like to do	$p<.01$	$p<.01$	$p<.001$	$p<.001$	$p<.001$
Judge their health as worse than five years ago	N.S.	$p<.001$	$p<.05$	N.S.	$p<.001$
Feel their work affects their health adversely	N.S.	N.S.	$p<.02$	N.S.	$p<.001$

(N.S. = Not Significant)

In their relationships with health professionals, the disadvantaged often reflect this desire for a transcendent exorcist, one who will perform specific, visible procedures on them, make decisions for them, and serve as a benign, confirming authority. Rural blacks, more than whites, want a physician who will offer much medication ($p<.001$) and agreement ($p<.001$). The less educated ($p<.05$, $p<.001$), the poor ($p<.05$, $p<.001$), and the emotionally impaired ($p<.001$, $p<.001$) express the same attitudes to an unusual degree. In addition, the poor desire a doctor who will make decisions for them ($p<.05$) more than do those persons with larger incomes.

The disadvantaged rural person expects less from treatment than do others. Blacks expect fewer cures ($p<.001$). The less educated and the poor believe that they get fewer cures ($p<.05$). The emotionally impaired expect cure less than partial measures. Far more than the unimpaired, they anticipate only partial recovery ($p<.05$), some retardation of illness ($p<.001$), a little relief from discomfort ($p<.001$) in contrast to full functionality. Parenthetically, it is surprising that only 11 percent of the overall sample expects any significant increase in understanding of their illness as a result of treatment.

While it is the current custom to speak of governmental agencies and insurance companies as the "third party" in health care payment plans, the disadvantaged see themselves as the passive third party in a transaction between two active participants: health professionals and insuring agencies. For example, blacks (when compared with whites) report less self-payment ($p<.05$) and add that they prefer other means of payment such as federal and state insurance ($p<.05$). If they pay, they are billed more often ($p<.001$) and prefer this method ($p<.001$) rather than payment at each visit. The same attitudes (at equal levels of significance) are expressed on all items by the elderly, the low education and income groups, and the emotionally impaired.

INTERPRETATION

The data above portray a constellation of attitudes held in common by those "set apart" in our society on the basis of their race, age, educational level, income, or emotional difficulties. This cluster of values is illuminated most vividly in rural areas, where the dimensions of deprivation stand out in bold relief. One would expect, however, to find similar views among the culturally deprived members of inner-city populations.

The study indicates that class, ethnic, and racial factors demarcate health attitudes more clearly than do sex factors. Membership in any of these groups has far-reaching effects upon the experiences and preferences of the individual. Participation in any socially deprived group makes one an "honorary member" of the larger subcommunity of the disadvantaged.

What are the "core" values cementing these groups? One explanation posits that the ultimate deprivation imposed by society is not the loss of money, learning, or youth. The greatest burden lies in the erosion of one's self-understanding as an effective, active agent, a legitimate and creative participant in social transactions (including health care). The socially disadvantaged have difficulty seeing themselves as initiators, asserters, colleagues in the delivery of health care. On the contrary, they see themselves as objects to be worked upon.

It is not surprising that they wait longer before seeking care, and then do so largely in acute situations (as one may neglect the maintenance of a machine or appliance, bringing it for repair only when it breaks down in a dramatic way). The disadvantaged seek powerful, transcendent healing figures as a reflection of their own sense of inadequacy to provide any significant biological, social, or economic contribution to the enhancement of their health. In like fashion, they expect little positive effect from treatment since they are unsure of their status as a resource or even as an object of worth. An additional expression of this self-perception is found in the disadvantaged patient's inability to conceive of himself as an active contributor financially. Herman alludes to this cluster of expectations:

> There are also a number of indications that the poor may less generally believe in the patient's responsibility to seek and follow professional advice, a widely held assumption among laymen of higher economic status and health professionals. However, only among the very poor and disorganized would these tendencies toward passivity and living in the present reach a state which could be called apathy or anomie.

Responsibility can be understood, not in a moralistic sense, but as "ability to respond." A person's sense of his worth and capacities is conferred in his interactions with significant others from early childhood onward. Mead has elaborated the insight that the world of the self is built "from the outside inward." That is, the growing person comes to see and value himself by taking the attitude of other people that he encounters as they observe him, respond to him, and judge him. The global, continual impact of negative responses to a person's ethnic, racial, or class status is a powerful shaping agent.

This is not to say that the disadvantaged become indifferent concerning the state of their health. Fifty-nine percent of poor blacks and 72 percent of poor whites in the country place good health above having a good job. This study does suggest that a culturally deprived person's self-understanding forms a complex, resistive pattern affecting his accessibility for health care, his utilization of health services, and his support of the health systems that serve him. The vicious cycle of depersonalizing reinforcement between poverty and illness is illustrated by the finding that low-income family members miss more days of work because of illness than do those with financial resources ($p < .05$). Absence from work due to illness leads to further depression of income and consequent increase in health problems. Both patterns damage the patient's sense of self-worth and constrict his health-seeking activity. Warheit reports that family income is the primary parameter differentiating deprived groups from others. When this factor is controlled statistically, the other variables studied (race, education, aging, emotional impairment) have decidedly less effect on health expectations.

A persistent question remains: "How shall health planners respond to the pervasive, depersonalizing self-understandings and consequent health attitudes of the disadvantaged?" Three alternatives require consideration:

1. Ignore these value patterns and their effects on health care efforts;
2. Accept and seek to justify the self-denigrating attitudes of culturally deprived patient populations;
3. Engage in a realistic, systematic attempt to alter the causes of such health expectations.

The first alternative, selective inattention, offers short-range relief from the anxieties that plague decision-makers in health systems. Administrators coping with the complexities of cost analysis, information storage, and manpower distribution resist additional grappling with the complicating attitudes of the poor or aging recipient. The overextended clinician is tempted to exclude the patient's expectations from the list of necessary ingredients in formulating a plan of care.

The second option, acceptance and legitimation of the patient's view of himself as a passive object, has appeal to the overworked, paternalistic "deliverer" of health care. It is easy to assume that disadvantaged patients are more comfortable (and therefore better served) when their self-demeaning roles are reinforced in the care setting. One must question whether such reinforcement is carried out to meet the security needs of the purveyor or the health needs of the consumer.

It is possible, of course, that the apathy and self-negation of rural disadvantaged patients may reflect realistic deficiencies in comparison to other populations. Many of the young, active, and better educated have left rural settings for the city. One might hypothesize that rural poverty may be a result of this social selection process rather than the primary cause of poor health attitudes. If the comparative study of rural and urban disadvantaged groups reveals differences of emotional, intellectual, and physical capability as well as attitude, then it would be reasonable to design health care reflecting these differences of capacity. In this case, the self-attitudes would be accepted as regrettably accurate. This approach, however, would require evidence of significant differences in the intrinsic resources of the rural deprived and other patient groups.

Ignoring or reinforcing disadvantaged patients' self-negating health attitudes can contribute to callousness among health professionals, jeopardize the effectiveness of care plans, and deepen the sense of alienation among those already culturally deprived. Under the twin pressures of shrinking financial support and enlarging demand for care, planners cannot afford to bypass patient value structures that hinder an effort demanding 7 percent of the gross national product. Further, disadvantaged patients who see themselves as nonproductive "consumers" will continue to consume welfare funds without contributing at all to the nation's economy. Through such self-limiting attitudes, the culturally deprived pass their poverty on to their peers and progeny.

Clearly, personnel must adjust the tactics of health care to those limiting health attitudes that defy change; the third alternative, however, seems both essential and promising. Every effort should be made to understand causes of deprived patients' constricting self-estimates and expectations. Increased knowledge of the sources of health attitudes may lead to a more flexible, effective range of health-seeking behavior.

Some social prescriptions for health care attitude change have been simplistic. The placing of "consumer representatives" from disadvantaged groups on health planning boards may neglect the fact that such participation cannot be more effective than the attitudes that such representatives bring to the planning process. Mechanic suggests another course: the establishment of medical ombudsmen, persons from disadvantaged populations who have received sufficient technical training to understand health care resources, methods, and issues. Although promising, this proposal raises difficult questions. How can we introduce the rural ombudsman to a sophisticated, academically centered, upper-middle-class world of health care delivery while ensuring his close relationship with the disadvantaged groups comprising his cultural home? What reward system (salary, fringe benefits, etc.) will give the ombudsman status and freedom in relationships with other health care providers without unfitting him to represent the deprived?

The use of economic measures to alter health attitudes is appealing. If level of family income is the primary factor differentiating the values of the deprived, will additional income alter these values? It is conceivable that the most effective changes in these self-constricting attitudes can be brought about by direct subsidies to the poor. On the other hand, this proposed solution neglects the consideration that both the low income and the self-defeating attitudes of the disadvantaged may be due to other causes (e.g., societal stereotypes regarding class, educational deprivation, early family influences, genetics, etc.).

The approaches mentioned above may be desirable, even necessary. Each alone is of doubtful sufficiency. In addition, research and teaching programs may assist health professionals and recipients to see the sources of patient values and their impact on the effectiveness of health care. Students in the health sciences can become acquainted, through clinical and course experiences, with the concepts and skills required for the effective care of the disadvantaged.

Whatever the methods employed, the goal is that of understanding and altering those values and behaviors that inhibit the creative health care of these socially deprived groups. The health professional should assist the poor, black, aging, undereducated, and emotionally impaired to gain a sense of realistic selfhood and a more effective range of health-seeking actions in a tragically limiting world.

In generalizing from rural to other disadvantaged subpopulations, one must be wary of overextending conclusions. Nevertheless, the membrane between rural and nonrural communities is a very porous one. The decisions of planners in urban settings have marked impact upon the countryside, and the reverberations of these effects are felt again in the city. With increased mobility and communication, rural youth form a large segment of the candidates for urban citizenship. They may bring with them the values characterized in this study. To use a sports analogy, the rural minor leagues still serve as a "farm system" for the development of the major league populations and issues confronting metropolitan America. Increased knowledge of the culturally deprived and their experiences may offer a clearer view of the options open to the health planner. In this fashion, the rural patient may hold a mirror up to his society, the aging may offer a legacy of new insight, the uneducated may provide new learnings, the poor, a wealth of understanding, and the estranged black person, a new foundation for the community.

VII. The Mental Health of a Rural County
An Epidemiologic Overview

George J. Warheit, Ph.D.

THE PURPOSE OF THIS CHAPTER is to describe and analyze some of the mental health characteristics of those included in the health study of Lafayette County, Florida. The analysis depends extensively on the use of the Leighton Health Opinion Survey (HOS), which has been used widely in a number of epidemiologic studies designed to evaluate the mental health of general populations.[1] Originally, many of the individual items in the HOS were part of the Army Neuropsychiatric Examination utilized during World War II by United States military health personnel. The present form of the HOS was developed and tested for reliability and validity by Alexander and Dorothea Leighton as part of their epidemiologic work on mental illness in Nova Scotia; their overall findings plus a discussion of the utility and limitations of the HOS have been reported in detail by them and their colleagues (cf. MacMillan, 1957). A number of others have tested the instrument for reliability and validity as well. Goldfarb et al. (1967a) documented the good interjudge reliability and repeat reliability of the HOS, and Goldfarb et al. (1967b) found that others could achieve acceptable reliability when compared to the Leightons' ratings. Moses et al. (1971) tested the instrument for validity and concluded that it was a useful device for determining the average level of psychopathology in one hundred active outpatients

1. A listing of the HOS items is found in the appendix to this chapter.

and a community sample of one hundred persons matched to the patients for age, sex, education, and marital status.

The HOS was tested for validity by Schwab and Warheit (1972), who administered the items to a random sample of 318 adults over age eighteen and 107 known psychiatric patients from the same general population. The 318 randomly selected respondents were then rated for social-psychiatric impairment by a panel of three psychiatrists; the ratings were based on written protocols which included an extensive inventory of physical and mental health items along with standard sociodemographic information such as age, race, sex, and so forth.[2] On the basis of extensive statistical analysis, they found that those rated as possible and probable cases had scores on the HOS significantly more similar to the patient groups than did the noncases.

In addition, Warheit and Hampton (1971) gathered HOS data on 528 adults as part of an in-depth evaluation of health needs and services in two central Florida counties. These adults, along with the 318 persons from the Schwab and Warheit pretest sample and the 1,645 respondents in their major study samples, provide a total of 2,491 adults for whom HOS scores have been obtained. This large number of randomly selected and personally interviewed adults constitutes a population base from which statistical norms for various sociodemographic groups in north and central Florida have been determined. These norms will be used for comparative analysis of the findings on the mental health characteristics of the Lafayette County sample.[3]

On the basis of these independent research efforts, it is reasonably safe to conclude that the HOS is both reliable and valid as a general screening instrument. It must be emphasized, however, that the HOS in its present form is not intended for use with individuals for diagnostic purposes, since it has not been tested sufficiently for validity and reliability for such use. It is also important to note that Schwab and Warheit discovered that 38.0 percent of the outpatients

2. The work of Schwab and Warheit reported here is from a pretest survey conducted as part of a major five-year study, "Evaluating Southern Mental Health Needs and Services." A report of their general pretest findings has been presented by them (Schwab and Warheit, 1972); a discussion of their concept of social-psychiatric impairment has also been published (Schwab et al., 1970).

3. Since the pretest has been completed, an additional 1,645 randomly selected respondents have been interviewed and are now being rated by three psychiatrists for social-psychiatric impairment. The Leighton caseness ratings on these additional 1,645 respondents have been determined and are listed as part of the normative distribution of Leighton scores reported in Table 1.

and 22.8 percent of the inpatients interviewed as part of their pretest study were found to be normal or "noncases" when rated by the scale score criteria (see Table 1). The reasons for this are not fully known, but it is suspected that the HOS does not detect many of the more severe psychotic symptoms, characterologic defects, or behavioral disorders. Its design more effectively detects psychoneurotic patterns and psychophysiologic symptoms; as such, conclusions about mental health and illness reached on the basis of the HOS must be

TABLE 1

LEIGHTON HOS MEAN SCORES AND CASENESS
RATINGS BY SAMPLE GROUPS

Sample	N	X	% Normal	% Possible Case	% Probable Case
County 1 pretest	318	28.0	74.9	18.5	6.6
County 1 main survey	1,643	27.0	74.5	16.4	9.2
Counties 2 & 3	528	26.8	74.8	14.9	10.2
% random sample rated impaired from pretest study	98	31.3	44.4	34.3	21.2
Psychiatric outpatients	50	33.0	38.0	28.0	34.0
Psychiatric inpatients	57	35.2	22.8	22.8	54.4
Lafayette Co.	126	31.1	50.8	25.4	23.8

interpreted carefully and in the light of these design characteristics. In spite of these limitations, there have been a sufficient number of independent research efforts to justify its use as a general measure of mental health and illness, particularly when the conclusions reached take into account the tendency of the HOS to focus on neuroticism and psychophysiologic symptomatology.

SCORING OF THE ITEMS

Researchers employing the HOS have used the scoring techniques developed by the Leightons. Those interviewed are asked to respond to the 20 questions on the basis of the frequency of occurrence of certain feelings or behaviors; the forced option choices are scored: 3 for "often," 2 for "sometimes," and 1 for "seldom or never." The scores are summed and the respondents assigned a probability of "caseness"[4] based on their total scores. The score criteria for caseness are as follows: 29 or under, not a case; 30–34, a possible case; and 35 and over, a probable case.

FINDINGS

The findings regarding the distribution of scores in Lafayette County are found in Table 1. The scores of respondents in three other Florida counties are also presented for purposes of comparison. The data show that the mean score of 31.1 for the Lafayette County sample was considerably higher than the average scores for the other counties. Significantly, the mean score for the Lafayette sample was almost identical to those rated as socially/psychiatrically impaired in the Schwab-Warheit pretest sample; moreover, the mean score of the Lafayette sample approached that of the Alachua County psychiatric outpatients, whose average score was 33.

When the data are translated into caseness ratings (Table 2), we find that only 50.8 percent of the total sample are classified as noncases, 25.4 percent are listed as possible cases, and 23.8 percent as probable cases. The analysis of caseness ratings by sociodemographic groups indicates that although more blacks than whites are rated as possible and probable cases, the overall differences are not statistically significant. The data on sex groups show a similar pattern; a higher percentage of females than males are possible or probable cases but the differences are not large enough to be statistically significant. The data on age indicate that older persons have higher rates of possible and probable caseness than the young; once again, however, the differences fall below the accepted levels for statistical significance.

The variations of caseness by family income are quite large; family income and caseness differences are statistically significant at the p < .001 level. Those having the highest levels of possible and probable caseness were found in the lowest family income groups. For example, 64.4 percent of those with annual family incomes of

4. By caseness, the Leightons mean that at some time in his adult life the respondent would qualify as a case according to the criteria of the 1952 Diagnostic and Statistical Manual of the American Psychiatric Association.

under $4,000 were either possible or probable cases, while none of those with family incomes over $8,000 were probable cases, and only 14.8 percent of this income group were possible cases.

The general pattern for educational achievement and caseness is an inverse one; the highest rates of caseness are found among those

TABLE 2

CASENESS RATINGS FOR TOTAL SAMPLE AND
SOCIODEMOGRAPHIC GROUPS BY PERCENTAGE
AND SIGNIFICANCE LEVELS

		Caseness			Significance Level
		Not a Case	Possible Case	Probable Case	X^2
Total sample	N-126	50.8	25.4	23.8	—
Race					
Black	N- 46	41.3	30.4	28.3	N.S.
White	N- 80	56.3	22.5	21.2	—
Sex					
Male	N- 49	59.2	18.4	22.4	N.S.
Female	N- 77	45.5	29.9	24.7	—
Age					
18–39	N- 36	58.3	30.6	11.1	N.S.
40–59	N- 43	55.8	20.9	23.3	—
60 and over	N- 47	40.4	25.5	34.0	—
Family income					
Under $4,000	N- 73	35.6	31.5	32.9	—
$4,000–$7,999	N- 24	58.3	16.7	25.0	p<.001
$8,000 and over	N- 27	85.2	14.8	0.0	—
Education					
Less than 4th grade	N- 28	28.6	28.6	42.9	p<.02
5–8th grade	N- 26	38.5	30.8	30.8	—
9–12th grade	N- 52	61.5	21.2	17.3	—
More than 12th grade	N- 19	73.7	21.1	5.3	—

with the least education and the lowest rates of caseness are among those with the highest educational achievement. The overall differences are statistically significant at the p < .02 level.

A more detailed statistical analysis is difficult because of the small sample. The percentages are indicative of certain trends, however, and these are worth noting. Table 3 presents the findings on caseness percentages by race and sex groupings. The data show that both black males and females have higher caseness ratings than their white counterparts; the data also reveal that females in both groups have a greater percentage of caseness than males. White males had the lowest percentage of caseness scores, black females the highest.

When the data are analyzed in terms of race, age, and caseness (Table 4), it is found that advancing age is associated with higher caseness ratings. The lowest percentages of possible and probable caseness in both races are among those under 40 years of age; those 60 years of age and over have very high rates of possible or probable

TABLE 3

PERCENTAGE OF CASENESS RATINGS
BY RACE AND SEX

| Race | | % Caseness Ratings | | |
		Not a Case	Possible Case	Probable Case
Black	N-46			
Male	N-12	50.0	16.7	33.3
Female	N-34	41.2	33.4	25.4
White	N-80			
Male	N-37	63.3	21.7	15.0
Female	N-43	54.5	27.1	18.4

caseness. Of the blacks 60 and over, 64.7 percent are found to be possible or probable cases; for whites in this age group, the total is 56.7 percent.

From the findings reported in Table 4, one might conclude that the race of the respondent is the major factor in accounting for possible or probable caseness. This, however, is not true, for when the data on caseness by race are controlled for family income (Table 5), one finds the differences between the two racial groups are practically nonexistent. Although the smallness of the sample, when divided by race, income, and caseness, limits the generalizability of the findings, the trends strongly suggest that family income and not race is the better predictor of possible or probable caseness.

These findings are generally consistent with the great majority of epidemiologic studies dealing with psychological-psychiatric disorders. Blacks, females, the aged, the poor, and those with limited educational achievement have the highest rates of possible or probable caseness, and, although the differences between the races, the

TABLE 4

PERCENTAGE OF CASENESS RATINGS
BY RACE AND AGE

		Not a Case	Possible Case	Probable Case
Blacks	N-46			
18–39	N-15	46.7	40.0	13.3
40–59	N-14	42.9	14.3	42.9
60 and over	N-17	35.3	35.3	29.4
Whites	N-80			
18–39	N-21	66.7	23.8	9.5
40–59	N-29	62.1	24.1	13.8
60 and over	N-30	43.3	20.0	36.7

sexes, and the various age groups were not found to be statistically significant, the percentage differences within these groups were often quite high and, as such, indicative of real differences in spite of their statistical shortcomings. The differences in caseness among the several income and education groups were highly significant. This finding of low socioeconomic status (as determined by income and education) is consistent with the forty-four epidemiologic studies of psychological disorder analyzed by the Dohrenwends (1969) and with those reported by Schwab and Warheit (1972) and Warheit and Hampton (1971) in their work in north and central Florida.

Economic factors may account for the very high rate of possible and probable caseness in the Lafayette County sample, in part, since there is a very low standard of living for many in the county. Even when socioeconomic factors are controlled, however, the rates of

TABLE 5

PERCENTAGE OF CASENESS RATINGS
BY RACE AND INCOME

		Not a Case	Possible Case	Probable Case
Blacks	N-45			
Under $4,000	N-39	33.0	33.3	33.3
$4,000–$7,999	N- 6	83.3	16.7	0.0
$8,000 and over	N- 0	0.0	0.0	0.0
Whites	N-79			
Under $4,000	N-34	38.2	29.4	32.4
$4,000–$7,999	N-18	50.0	16.7	33.3
$8,000 and over	N-27	85.2	14.8	0.0

caseness are considerably higher than in County 1 where 53.6 percent of those with annual incomes of under $3,000 were possible or probable cases, or in Counties 2 and 3 where 39.7 percent of this same income category were in the caseness groups. What may be occurring is that the HOS items, which are designed in part to identify the presence of psychophysiological symptoms, are detecting high rates of somatic complaints and physical illnesses, which are widespread in the county's population. A more detailed discussion of these questions is presented in the concluding section of this chapter. In an effort to put the caseness findings in a broader health perspective, we have analyzed the caseness groups in terms of their self-perception of general health, the patterns of health and illness within their families, and their degree of functional loss.

SUBJECTIVE PERCEPTIONS OF HEALTH IN GENERAL

The findings which relate the respondent's subjective feelings regarding his physical health and the caseness percentages by response groups are reported in Table 6. The question asked was: ''How would you say that your health in general has been?'' The forced option answers were good, medium, and poor. As shown in Table 6, there is a high association between the subjective perception of the respondents' physical health and their caseness percentages; those who said their health in general was either poor or medium were far more likely to have scores in the caseness ranges than those who rated their health as good. Of the fifty-seven whites who reported their health as good, 73.7 percent had scores in the noncase category; for the twenty-one blacks who said their health in general was good, 81.0 percent had scale scores in the noncase range. By contrast, 66.6 percent of the whites who reported their health as poor were probable cases and 16.7 percent were possible cases; for blacks who said their health was poor, 90.9 percent were in the probable case category and 9.1 percent were in the possible case range. When the data on those reporting their health as medium are analyzed, one finds that 90.9 percent of the whites and 85.7 percent of the blacks who reported their health as medium had scores which identified them as possible or probable cases. Very obviously, there is a strong association between the self-perception of health in general and the likelihood of being rated a case on the basis of HOS scores. Of those reporting on their health in general, only those rating it as good were likely to be

TABLE 6

CASENESS PERCENTAGES BY RESPONDENTS' SELF-PERCEPTION
OF PHYSICAL HEALTH—CONTROLLED FOR RACE

Perception of Health by Caseness Categories	Racial Groups by Caseness Percentages	
Good	White (N-57)	Black (N-21)
Not a case	73.7	81.0
Possible	17.5	19.0
Probable	8.8	0.0
Medium	White (N-11)	Black (N-14)
Not a case	9.1	14.3
Possible	54.5	64.3
Probable	36.4	21.4
Poor	White (N-12)	Black (N-11)
Not a case	16.7	0.0
Possible	16.7	9.1
Probable	66.6	90.9

noncases. The responses to this question alone appear to serve as a powerful predictor of caseness as judged by the Leighton Survey.

When the data on the utilization of health care facilities are presented (Table 7), it is found that the health-care-seeking behavior of the various caseness groups is markedly different. Interestingly, those in the noncase category used the services of the Health Center in the county more often than did the caseness groups; about three-fourths of the noncase respondents reported they were clinic users, whereas slightly more than one-half of those in the caseness groups indicated such use. As far as clinic utilization is concerned, the possible and probable groups are more similar to one another than either is to the noncase group. When the data on hospitalizations in

TABLE 7

PERCENTAGE OF CASENESS GROUPS REPORTING
UTILIZATION OF HEALTH CLINIC HOSPITAL

Caseness Groups		% Using Clinic	% Hospitalized in Last Year
Not a case	(N-64)	70.0	19.8
Possible case	(N-32)	56.1	18.9
Probable case	(N-30)	56.6	50.0

the last year are reviewed, however, a different pattern is seen. Just slightly less than 20 percent of those in the noncase and possible case groups reported being hospitalized in the year prior to the interview, while 50 percent of the probable case group reported at least one hospitalization. Thus, the noncase group reported using the clinic more frequently than either of the case groups but those in the probable case group reported more hospitalizations. From this one can conclude that perhaps those in the noncase group seek health care earlier and / or on a more routine basis than those listed as cases, and further that those with the greatest probability of caseness either do not seek routine health care or delay treatment until hospitalization becomes necessary.

In summary, the data reported in Tables 6 and 7 indicate that (1) the caseness groups view their health less favorably than the noncase group, (2) the case groups use the clinic facilities less often than the noncase group, and (3) those most likely to be cases report more than two times the percentage of hospitalizations than those in the possible and noncase categories.

PATTERNS OF FAMILY HEALTH

The patterns of illness among family members of the three caseness groups is an alternating one. As shown in Table 8, those most likely to be cases are from family situations where illness and disability are commonplace. Among the probable case group, 60 percent reported the presence of physical illness among other family members, 36.6 percent indicated that some member of the family (other than themselves) had some physical disability, and 56.6 percent said there were family members who had emotional or mental health problems. The possible case group reported percentages of physical illness and disability among other family members at about the same level as the noncase group; about one-fourth of these two groups indicated that there were family members with physical health problems and from 6 to 11 percent reported disability among other family members. Interestingly, however, 46.9 percent of the possible case group said there were others in their families who had mental or emotional problems, while 20.3 percent of those in the noncase group reported similar problems. Thus, while the noncase and possible case groups report like percentages of physical illness and disability among other family members, the two caseness groups reported far higher and more similar percentages of other family members with mental or emotional problems. It is important to note, also, that even the noncase group reported a relatively high percentage of family members with mental or emotional problems, 20.3 percent; this percentage is almost twice as high as those in this group reporting family disability,10.9 percent, and approximately equal to the percentage reporting physical health problems, 23.4 percent. These subjective reports by the respondents strongly suggest that mental and emotional problems are present in many of the households in the county; 33.3 percent of the total sample reported the existence of such problems.

TABLE 8

PERCENTAGE OF CASENESS GROUPS REPORTING HEALTH
PROBLEMS OF OTHER FAMILY MEMBERS

Problem	Not a Case (N-64)	Possible Case (N-32)	Probable Case (N-30)
Physical problems of other family member	23.4	21.8	60.0
Disability of other family member	10.9	6.3	36.6
Mental / emotional problem of other family member	20.3	46.9	56.6

FUNCTIONAL LOSS AND CASENESS

The data found in Tables 9 and 10 demonstrate the dramatic differences in the amount of functional loss encountered by the various caseness groups. Significantly, the relationship between the number of days of work missed and caseness (Table 9) is a direct one. Eighty percent of those in the probable case group reported they missed two or more weeks from their routine work during the year prior to the interview; this compares to 33.3 percent for the possible case and 14.3 percent for the noncase groups. In addition to the question dealing with the loss of work, three other questions which deal with functional loss were asked the respondents. These were "Have you ever

TABLE 9

AMOUNT OF TIME MISSED FROM ROUTINE WORK AS THE RESULT
OF ILLNESS BY CASENESS GROUPS
(in percentages)

| Caseness Groups | | Days Missed | |
		None or a Few Days	Two Weeks or More
Not a case	(N-64)	85.7	14.3
Possible case	(N-32)	66.6	33.3
Probable case	(N-30)	20.0	80.0

TABLE 10

PERCENTAGE OF FUNCTIONAL LOSS
REPORTED BY CASENESS GROUPS

Caseness Groups		Often	Sometimes, Seldom	Never
Have you ever had to go easy on work because of poor health?				
Not a case	(N-64)	4.7	45.3	50.0
Possible case	(N-32)	9.1	59.8	31.1
Probable case	(N-30)	50.0	50.0	0.0
Have you ever had periods of days, weeks, or months when you couldn't get going?				
Not a case	(N-64)	4.7	61.2	34.1
Possible case	(N-32)	21.6	68.8	9.6
Probable case	(N-30)	60.0	36.6	3.4
Do you feel healthy enough to carry out the things you would like to do?				
Not a case	(N-64)	89.1	6.2	4.7
Possible case	(N-32)	53.1	46.9	0.0
Probable case	(N-30)	18.7	62.6	18.7

had to go easy on your work because of poor health? Have you ever had periods of days, weeks, or months when you couldn't get going? Do you feel healthy enough to carry out the things you would like to do?" The last of these items is part of the HOS; consequently, one would expect those in the caseness categories to have larger percentages of negative responses to this question than those in the noncase group. The tautological nature of this item is recognized, but it is reported here because it represents part of a syndrome of functional loss on the part of the caseness groups. The responses to this item are reversed from the other ones dealing with function; in this instance the negative responses are suggestive of pathology.

A close examination of the findings reported in Table 10 reinforces those found in Table 9: there is a definite relationship between possible and probable caseness and functional loss measured in behavioral terms. Those in the caseness categories reported far more often that they had to go easy on work, that for prolonged periods they could not get going, and that they frequently did not feel healthy enough to carry out the things they wanted to do. The responses to these questions indicate clearly that those having HOS scores in the caseness ranges reported far more functional impairment than those in the noncase group.

One can probably assume that these functional limitations not only impede these individuals in the performance of their work roles but limit the fulfillment of other social roles as well, and, importantly, limit them in the possibilities of attaining a full and satisfying life.

SUMMARY AND CONCLUSIONS

The purpose of this chapter has been to describe the mental health characteristics of a sample of persons living in a rural county in northwest Florida. The Health Opinion Survey, developed by Alexander and Dorothea Leighton and their colleagues, was used as the primary rating instrument by which the sample was categorized into three caseness groups: noncases, possible cases, and probable cases. The findings on caseness for Lafayette County were compared with those of 2,491 persons from three other counties in north and central Florida. The Lafayette sample had substantially more persons in it with possible and probable caseness ratings than did the other three counties; 49.2 percent of the Lafayette group were rated as possible or probable cases compared to about 25 percent in the other samples.

The mean score on the HOS for the Lafayette County sample was 31.3 percent; this is very close to the mean score of a group of randomly selected respondents from a related study, who were rated as socially / psychiatrically impaired by three psychiatric raters and compared to the mean score of 33 percent for a group of known psychiatric outpatients.

When the data were analyzed by sociodemographic groups, it was found that blacks, females, the elderly, the poor, and the least educated had the highest rates of caseness. The differences between blacks and whites, males and females, and the young and old were not found to be statistically significant; the difference between caseness groups by family income was statistically significant at the p<.001 level and the differences in educational level and caseness were significant at the p<.02 level. The data on caseness by race indicated no significant differences between the races when controlled for family income.

The caseness groups saw their health as being worse than the noncase group; they used the services of the Lafayette County Health Center less often, but those in the probable case category reported a far higher percentage of hospitalizations than the noncase and possible case groups. Those with probable case ratings reported most often that there were other family members with physical and mental health problems; both caseness groups reported much higher percentages of other family members suffering from mental or emotional problems than did the noncase group. The caseness groups also reported much higher levels of functional impairment as measured by time missed from routine work, going easy on work, not being able to get going, and not feeling healthy enough to carry out the things they would like to do.

These findings, when seen from a total perspective, form a configuration which is unmistakable. The population of Lafayette County has inordinately high rates of caseness as judged by the Leighton HOS. The possible sources of explanation of these high rates are both methodological and theoretical. At the methodological level, it can be argued that these high rates of caseness among residents of the county are due to the confounding of mental and physical symptomatology by the HOS. Since the survey contains a number of items designed to detect psychophysiologic symptomatology, it can be contended that the high rates of caseness are an artifact of the survey instrument, which is detecting the somatic complaints and illnesses of an economically and medically deprived group of people and confounding them in terms of mental health problems.

While this argument undoubtedly contains elements of truth, it raises another fundamental question: namely, can one really dichotomize physical and mental health into separate categories? The answer is probably no. In reality these two dimensions of health are so highly interrelated that they are all but inseparable, except, perhaps, by heuristic definitions designed to aid the scientist or clinician in his work. A full discussion of this issue is beyond the immediate scope of this chapter and will not be discussed in further detail; our not dealing with it more extensively is not intended to deny its importance or the fact that the high rates of physical symptomatology are undoubtedly related to the high rates of caseness on the Leighton HOS.

At a more theoretical level, our data, which indicate that the highest rates of mental health problems are found among the lowest socioeconomic groups, are relevant to the testing of an experiment proposed by Dohrenwend and Dohrenwend (1969). They suggest a procedure which enables researchers to test the relative importance of the two major hypotheses offered most often as possible explanations of this recurring phenomenon: social selection and social causality. Briefly stated, the social causation thesis suggests that low social status produces psychopathology; the social selection position asserts that pre-existing disorders determine low socioeconomic status. The Dohrenwends indicate that the social causation hypothesis can be tested most effectively by comparing the rates of disorder among persons in advantaged and disadvantaged groups after they have been controlled for social class. The argument is that if the rates of disorder are higher in the disadvantaged groups, even when controlled for key social class indicators such as income and education, a strong argument can be made for the social causation position. The reasoning is that increased downward social pressure on disadvantaged persons would produce greater psychopathology than that produced by the lesser downward social pressures on the more advantaged groups.

On the other hand, if one finds, after controlling for social class, that the rates among the disadvantaged groups are lower than their class counterparts in the advantaged groups, the implication would be that class differences in the rates of disorder are due more to social selection than social causation. One could argue the validity of this in that the lower rates of disorder among the disadvantaged groups demonstrate that downward social pressure does not lead to increased psychopathology but rather these pressures tend to block the upward social mobility of healthy members of the disadvantaged group more than that of the psychologically healthy members of advantaged groups. These social selection processes would "sort out" a larger number of ill among the low status persons in the advantaged groups, who would form a residual population of highly impaired persons.

The empirical question is if blacks in our sample have higher or lower rates of caseness than whites, when social class factors are controlled. The answer is equivocal, since our finding is that when social class factors are controlled, there are no significant differences in the rates of the two racial groups. Thus, it is impossible to accept either of the hypotheses as posited by the Dohrenwends. What the data suggest specifically is that (1) there are no statistically significant differences between the advantaged (white) group and the disadvantaged (black) group, when social class factors are held constant; thus, the social selection argument cannot be accepted, since the low status whites do not have higher rates of caseness than low status blacks, and (2) the social causation position as outlined by the Dohrenwends cannot be accepted or rejected since the rates for both groups are the same. Had the rates been higher for blacks than whites, when controlled for socioeconomic status, a strong argument could have been made for social causation. On the other hand, had the rates been lower for blacks than whites, the implications would have pointed toward social selection.

Thus, our findings as related to the experiment offered by the Dohrenwends are inconclusive. The data suggest that if lower social status is causally related to high rates of caseness, its impact is approximately equal in seriously disadvantaged groups, regardless of racial origin.

The inability to establish, definitively, a causal relationship between social class factors and high rates of caseness in terms of social selection and social causation does not prevent us from concluding what is quite obvious: there is a high relationship between socioeconomic factors and health, be it labeled physical or mental. The implications for those delivering health care to this residual population, and to countless others similar to it in terms of age, sex, race, socioeconomic, and geographic factors, are evident. The health needs of these populations are immense, and they include the necessity of treating the whole person; to emphasize physical health care at the neglect of mental health services will diminish the effectiveness of the health care givers and the system within which they function.

APPENDIX

HEALTH OPINION SURVEY

The Twenty Questions

1. Do you have any physical or health problems at the present?
   Yes (3)   No (1)
2. Do your hands ever tremble enough to bother you?
   Often (3)   Sometimes (2)   Never (1)
3. Are you ever troubled by your hands or feet sweating so that they feel damp and clammy?
   Often (3)   Sometimes (2)   Never (1)
4. Have you ever been bothered by your heart beating hard?
   Often (3)   Sometimes (2)   Never (1)
5. Do you tend to feel tired in the mornings?
   Often (3)   Sometimes (2)   Never (1)
6. Do you have any trouble getting to sleep and staying asleep?
   Often (3)   Sometimes (2)   Never (1)
7. How often are you bothered by having an upset stomach?
   Often (3)   Sometimes (2)   Never (1)
8. Are you ever bothered by nightmares (dreams which frighten you)?
   Often (3)   Sometimes (2)   Never (1)
9. Have you ever been troubled by "cold sweats"?
   Often (3)   Sometimes (2)   Never (1)
10. Do you feel that you are bothered by all sorts (different kinds) of ailments in different parts of your body?
    Often (3)   Sometimes (2)   Never (1)
11. Do you smoke?
    A lot (3)   Some (2) Not at all (1)
12. Do you ever have loss of appetite?
    Often (3)   Sometimes (2)   Never (1)
13. Has any ill health affected the amount of work (housework) you do?
    Often (3)   Sometimes (2)   Never (1)
14. Do you ever feel weak all over?
    Often (3)   Sometimes (2)   Never (1)
15. Do you ever have spells of dizziness?
    Often (3)   Sometimes (2)   Never (1)
16. Do you tend to lose weight when you worry?
    Often (3)   Sometimes (2)   Never (1)
17. Have you ever been bothered by shortness of breath when you were not exerting yourself?
    Often (3)   Sometimes (2)   Never (1)
18. For the most part, do you feel healthy enough to carry out the things that you would like to do?
    Often (1)   Sometimes (2)   Never (3)

19. Do you feel in good spirits?

Most of the time (1)   Sometimes (2)   Very few
                                                                     times (3)

20. Do you sometimes wonder if anything is worthwhile anymore?

Often (3)   Sometimes (2)   Never (1)

With the scores assigned to the above responses, the higher the total score, the greater the likelihood of psychoneurotic disorder. (Note the reversed order of response weights in questions 18 and 19.) It is highly desirable that the respondent should be required to select one, and only one, of the scorable responses.

20–29 NOT A CASE
30–34 POSSIBLE CASE
35 +   PROBABLE CASE

As an example of how the score for an individual is determined, consider the following possible responses:

QUESTION	RESPONSE	SCORE	QUESTION	RESPONSE	SCORE
1	No	1	11	A lot	3
2	Sometimes	2	12	Sometimes	2
3	Often	3	13	Never	1
4	Sometimes	2	14	Never	1
5	Often	3	15	Never	1
6	Never	1	16	Sometimes	2
7	Never	1	17	Sometimes	2
8	Never	1	18	Never	3
9	Sometimes	2	19	Very few times	3
10	Often	3	20	Sometimes	2

Sum of scores = 39

The mean score of the sample, or any subgrouping, would be the sum of the individuals' scores divided by the number in the sample or subgrouping.

For those who are interested in the historical development of this instrument, a detailed and technical memorandum is available for the asking.

VIII. Folk Beliefs
Understanding of Health, Illness, and Treatment

Alice H. Murphree, M.A.

ALTHOUGH THE LITERATURE seems to lack specific definitions for "folk belief," abundant descriptions ensure a general understanding of the term. Here, the term will be used to refer to widely accepted views and opinions based on empirical experiences. Drawn from a common pool of knowledge about specific situations or things, folk beliefs serve as the basis for judgments and consequent coping behavior.[1]

The term "folk belief " frequently evokes an image of curious, interestingly esoteric attitudes and practices. Such an image is, in part, accurate; however, a much more comprehensive significance is associated with the term. Based on empirical experiences, judgments always have been made and are continuing to appear concerning appropriate behavior in any given situation. Such judgments apply to health and to all other aspects of life.

One proposition of the present discussion is that folk beliefs and practices are as contemporary as they are historical. To approach substantiation of this proposition, an examination of the formative process involved in folk beliefs and practices seems appropriate. Such an examination of this process relative to health beliefs in a rural community of the South will be a major theme in this chapter.

1. Portions of this chapter are expansions of a paper, "I've Come to Get a Shot: Contemporary Folk Belief in Process," presented at the Proceedings of the Southern Anthropological Society, February 1972, in Columbia, Missouri.

Also, folk beliefs, and resultant practices, are directly related to and expressive of any given cultural setting. Thus, they may reflect and be applied to any aspect of daily living. A study of folk remedies can provide valid indices of attitudes toward health and life itself. Folk beliefs may be analyzed in a vertical framework, historically over time, or they may be conceptualized horizontally within contemporary relationships with other facets of culture. Both approaches are fruitful and necessary and will be used in this presentation.

A brief review of the general characteristics of Lafayette County, as detailed in Chapter II, should provide background for the following discussion. Agriculture and forestry dominate the relatively constricted economy, and local resources for problem solving are sparse. This rural population typifies the social features of a residual group as it is small, relatively stable, and age skewed. Interpersonal relationships are predominantly primary: daily face-to-face interactions are among individuals well known (or even related) to each other. Because of long-term stability, the marriage patterns have produced an extremely intricate kinship system; there is a ring of validity in the common assertion, "Ever'body's kin to ever'body 'round here." The tenets of nineteenth century Protestantism dominate the value system, and church affiliations and associations play a major role in most people's lives. Change, in almost any sphere, comes with marked slowness; in fact, that which is new to the scene (including people) is, by definition, subject to suspicion.

THE RESEARCH

The data on which this discussion is based result from two specific field-work projects and a continuing, less formally structured study of health resources and utilization in Lafayette County. Included is a specific concern with folk medicine. For the first base-line study, the households of eighth-grade school children and some of their grandparental households were used.[2] There were fifty-four eighth-grade and sixteen grandparental households. In addition to the seventy base households, there were thirty-five individual interviews with school personnel, businessmen, governmental and political officials,

2. Murphree, 1965a.

representatives of the health fields, and key informants for "ole timey" remedies.

Health information sheets were administered to the eighth graders at the schools, and open-ended-question interviews were conducted in the households and elsewhere. As appropriate, brief mnemonic notes were taken during interviews and observations. Detailed field notes, both direct and impressional, were recorded immediately following each field experience. Evaluation and analysis were ongoing and finally were completed upon return from the field.

In the initial study, emphasis was on general statements about health conditions, past and present self-reported illnesses, number and site of hospitalizations, identification of physicians visited, reasons for seeking orthodox health assistance, dental care, and utilization of other health resources. Observations were made in the households, on the farms, in "the woods," in offices, schools, public places of work and recreation, and along the roads and highways of the county. The intensive field work was completed during six months, with several subsequent visits to validate and further cross-check data.

The second structured study was to research self-treatment practices, physician dependence, and the extent to which patients reveal to their physicians their self-treatment practices. During approximately eight months, two sets of interviews were conducted —one with Lafayette County residents and the other with their physicians in neighboring towns. With the exception of school health information sheets, the field methods outlined above were used again. There were eighty-eight randomized households, no households of the previous study being reinterviewed. Again, key informants were utilized for validation and cross-checking.

The less formally structured research has extended over a period of four years in connection with the establishment and operation of the teaching outpatient clinic in Lafayette County. This has included continuing interactions with county residents, plus those with students, staff, faculty, and visiting representatives of various agencies and institutions at the clinic. There has been the added dimension of viewing the county residents as patients and utilizers (or nonutilizers) of the clinic. The research role has been expanded to cover liaison between the community and the clinic and, at times, mutual interpretation.

EMERGING PATTERNS

Several pertinent patterns have emerged as a result of the research. Given the characteristics of a residual population, one such pattern is the marked introspection and self-concern found both in individuals and in the group. The introversion, combined with the strong religious influence and the effects of education, economics, and livelihood activities, results in a significant expression of concrete, cause-and-effect attitudes. As applied to health, this is reflected in acute somatic concern for such functions as digestion, elimination, or "nerves." Again, significantly, various "nervous" complaints are considered of somatic, rather than of emotional, etiology. Further expression of concreteness may be found in the literal interpretation of patent medicine television commercials, which frequently are used to describe symptoms and for self-diagnosis and consequent self-treatment.

Another pattern of the mechanistic understanding of physiology, expressed by such comments as the "coating on the nerves," accounts for various health conditions. The nervous system is apparently viewed as almost precisely duplicating an electrical system using insulated wires, the condition of the insulation being tied directly to the degree of illness or health. The cause-and-effect orientation similarly operates in the common, religion-related belief that illness is punishment for wrongdoing and good health is somewhat a reward for virtue. The concrete, cause-and-effect thinking is also manifested in the homeopathic and contagious magic of the several conjures in the actual folk medicine practices.

Two of the most relevant characteristics of folk beliefs are their dynamic quality and the fact that, by their adherents, folk beliefs and scientific medicine are *not* held to be mutually exclusive. Commonly, folk medicine may be used in lieu of, or simultaneously with, prescriptions. A third characteristic is tenacity. Because of its traditional nature, folk belief is familiar and comfortable and, in many contemporary instances, less expensive than physicians' treatment regimens. The entire formal medical milieu may be unfamiliar, uncomfortable, and frightening. Because it is common knowledge, also, that orthodox medicine tends to denigrate folk beliefs, denial of those beliefs or practices is similarly common. In nonthreatening situations, however, "ole timey" remedies and cures can be the theme of lively, productive conversations. Many reminiscences and experiences of rural residents are exchanged and discussed among themselves, thus substantiating efficacy.

Closely related to the dynamic quality are the adaptability and pervasiveness of folk beliefs. Practices based on intangibles may be transmitted virtually intact from generation to generation and from place to place. Those not completely suitable for a new time or new location can be modified. When new situations give rise to new needs, new folk solutions can be found.

To summarize an indication of the prevalence of folk belief in Lafayette County, the following data may be pertinent. As reported elsewhere (Murphree 1965a, 1968; Murphree and Barrow, 1970) during the original base-line study of 70 Lafayette County households, 221 different remedies were recorded, among which were 56 remedies using 40 species of plants. In the second study using 88 stratified random sample households, 11 percent of the respondents admitted current use and 70 percent acknowledged past use of folk medicines, while 27 percent were able to supply at least one specific recipe or verbal formula. As shown in Table 1, there were 66 references to folk medicine for 31 different complaints.

Few of the beliefs or practices collected in this research were specific to race; rather, most of them seem to be shared. Several are recognizably very old. Certainly, the dominance patterns of "sides" concerning some birth beliefs date back at least to ancient Greece; this is associated with the belief that the right side of the body is the masculine and the left side is the feminine. It may stem from the feeling that the right hand is stronger than the left, and males are considered stronger physically than females. The folk belief is expressed in such commonly repeated statements as the following: The foot with which a pregnant woman steps into a car or begins climbing steps indicates the sex of her unborn child—right for males and left for females. It must be remembered that the white settlers of Lafayette County and its environs brought their folk beliefs from other parts of the New World and, prior to that, from northern Europe. The blacks brought theirs from the Caribbean or elsewhere in the South and, previously, from Africa.

Those beliefs involving religious aspects required little, if any, modification—religious beliefs can function in almost any physical setting. One example is the use, by one who "has his mind on the Lord," of a Bible verse, Ezekiel 16:6 ("And when I passed by thee, and saw thee polluted in thine own blood, I said unto thee when thou

TABLE 1

FREQUENCY OF REFERENCES TO FOLK TREATMENTS
FOR SPECIFIC COMPLAINTS

Complaints	Frequency of References
Arthritis	1
Bleeding	2
Chills and fever	5
Colds	6
Colic	1
Cramping	1
Diabetes mellitus	2
Diarrhea	1
Erysipelas	1
Gallbladder	1
High blood (pressure)	1
Hives	3
Infection	3
"Low blood" or "run down" (anemia)	4
Malaria	3
Measles	3
Miscarriage	1
Pain	1
Piles	1
Rheumatism	1
"Risin's" (boils)	3
Ringworm	1
Sore eyes (conjunctivitis)	2
Sprains	3
Stomach trouble, nervous stomach, upset stomach, vomiting	6
Teething	2
"Thrash" (thrush)	1
Toothache	1
Warts	2
Whooping cough	2
Worms	1
Total	66

wast in thy blood, Live: yea, I said unto thee when thou wast in thy blood, Live.") as the verbal formula to "stop blood" (control excessive bleeding). This "cure," widely known in Lafayette County, is cited in the literature from other parts of the United States and from Europe. This particular belief exemplifies not only the transportability of folklore but also the literal, functionalistic interpretation of the

Bible, so commonly found in rural America and elsewhere. That
verse, out of context of the chapter, is appropriately worded for its
application to blood loss. Considered in terms of the entire chapter,
however, there is little to recommend it for this purpose. Here, too,
we find expression of the concreteness of attitudes.

Other verbal formulas to "stop blood" or "talk the fire out of a
burn" which invoke the Christian deities also have wide recognition
in Lafayette County. In addition, there are at least two conjures for
curing "the thrash" (thrush)—the fungus infection of the oral cavity
of children that impedes nursing. Here, however, in at least one of the
conjures, the leaf of a plant is used. If the traditionally required plant
did not grow in north Florida, a substitution from the local flora could
have been made, while retaining the original verbal formula.

It is also generally acknowledged that only people with "the
power" are able to effect such cures and conjures. It is generally
"known," also, that to maintain one's power, precise folk-curing
instruction can be transmitted only cross-sexually, outside the nu-
clear family. In other words, a woman cannot talk about her power
with another woman, nor a man with a man.

Those "ole timey" remedies utilizing household materials,
common to any setting, would be as easy to transport intact as are the
verbal formulas. The use of a sharp instrument, placed under the
pillow, mattress, or bed, to "cut" labor or afterbirth pains is an
example—and note the concreteness. What household did (or does)
not have a knife, scissors, razor, or axe? Likewise, few households
are without salt—for use in hot solution to soak aching muscles, or to
be given, one teaspoonful on three successive mornings, to a favorite
hunting dog suffering from distemper.

The practice of using chickens, or their blood, for prevention or
treatment of chicken pox illustrates homeopathic qualities of "like for
like" and, again, transportability. Neither domesticated chickens nor
the disease chicken pox were indigenous to the New World. Hence,
the source for this practice must have been Europe or Africa
via the Caribbean. One might tend to favor the latter because
chickens play a prominent part in much of the Caribbean voodoo lore.

Turning now to remedies using plants, we find that more adaptation may have been necessary. Many involve plant species found
both in Europe and in North America. A drop of "roasted out" onion
juice for earache could be a remnant of European or Eastern heritage.

Similarly, the use of wilted cabbage or turnip leaves, to "draw out the poison" from an infected cut, may not necessarily be a New World introduction into the folklore; however, a warm climate must have been the original source for using a prickly pear (a cactus) poultice to treat slow-healing "risin's," sores, or cuts. This latter could have come from the Mediterranean area, Africa, or from the New World.

In contrast, the use of plants indigenous to the New World strongly suggests American Indian contributions, or at least imitation or experimental discovery by whites or blacks. To eat raw sweet potato to "stop the stomach from running off" (diarrhea) or to drink corn shuck tea to "break out" the measles or to clear congestion and "run down the fever" in pneumonia are American in origin. Sweet potatoes and corn are New World plants.

Not all folk beliefs have their roots in the distant past, however; the dynamic process associated with folk beliefs is also found in a very contemporary phenomenon. The following vignette describes what has come to be a relatively frequent occurrence in many health care facilities and has been common in the teaching clinic in Lafayette County.

A patient arrives announcing, "I've come to get a penicillin shot, because I have a sore throat," or ". . . a bad cold," or ". . . the flu." The physician, or other health care personnel, ex- amines the patient and various diagnostic procedures are per- formed. During the evaluation, the patient becomes increasingly agitated and may comment, "I don't need all this—just give me my shot and let me get out of here." The evaluation indicates an infection of viral, rather than bacterial, etiology. Carefully, it is explained to the patient that, barring unforeseen complications, the illness is benign and will be of short duration. He is told that an antibiotic shot not only will not help him but may be harmful, as often there are dangerous physical reactions from such medi- cation. Appropriate treatment procedures are presented and their use firmly urged. The patient responds with hostility, if not anger, and stalks out stating, "I want a penicillin shot! I'll go see a *real* doctor who knows what he is doing!" The staff is aware that the directions for illness management well may be ignored.

The patient has self-diagnosed his illness and formulated a treatment regime including self-prescription. He, or she, strongly believes his is the better treatment course and cannot accept alternate prescriptions or treatment plans, despite the fullness of attempted explanations. He is convinced "a shot" of penicillin will afford almost immediate comfort and will effect a rapid cure. Although in different circumstances, patients request other injections such as B_{12}, here we will be concerned only with the more frequently requested antibiotic injections.

Penicillin was discovered in 1929, but it was not until the 1940s, circa World War II, that the advent of injectible penicillin initiated a widespread utilization of this treatment modality. In both medical and popular literature, antibiotics were heralded as quick-acting "miracle drugs," commonly associated with the progressive, scientific age. At the present time, at least two generations have been so treated. Virology was a routine part of medical education by the early 1950s. Research continued, and among the results were two facts: unlike pathogenic bacterial organisms, viral organisms do *not* respond to penicillin, and the majority of viral infections are self-limiting. Subsequently, clinical and laboratory data further indicated possible severe or even life-threatening reactions from some antibiotics. By the mid-fifties, these additional data were also being disseminated in medical and popular media. The more recent information to the contrary, the belief persists in Lafayette County and elsewhere that "a shot" of penicillin will most effectively treat many, but particularly respiratory, diseases.

The shot syndrome has been observed in numerous geographic areas. As personal observation of it has been restricted to rural, north central Florida, however, the present discussion pertains only to that particular setting. It is suggested that the attitude concerning shots is tenacious enough to qualify as an incipient folk belief. That postulate will be analyzed and the related sex role models will be considered.

Referring to the previous definition of folk belief, what were the empirical experiences associated with penicillin shots? And how did they relate to rural southern values? Injections, per se, had been familiar since the decade of the twenties. They had effectively immunized against, and hence controlled, such well-known and much-feared diseases as diphtheria and typhoid fever. For instance, by World War II most, if not all, southerners were customarily taking the routine three-injection immunization series and the annual booster shots for typhoid. Incidentally, in local idiom, currently there tends to be a three-way synonymous linkage among "shots," "penicillin shots," and "antibiotic shots."

For approximately the first decade of their use, penicillin injections were widely administered. They could be given quickly and, if necessary, by paramedical personnel. Men returning to rural civilian communities had vivid memories of their successful use by the military medical corps. In the busy rural practices (and these areas long have had a disproportionate ratio of physicians to population), physicians eagerly grasped the injectible antibiotics to increase the number of treatments delivered in a given period of time. It became common knowledge that "All doctors give penicillin shots."

Initially, there was only rudimentary information about the self-limiting characteristics of the viral infections. Consider the dynamics of the patient's experience as he sought medical attention with his inadequate understanding of viral infections. He was sick and received a penicillin injection. If the illness was a bacterially caused infection, it usually responded to the treatment, and the patient experienced rapid relief of symptoms and was well. If the illness resulted from a self-limiting virus, the patient also recovered quickly. Inability to differentiate the etiologies of his illnesses was the crux of the matter.

The effects of penicillin injections were obvious. Such commonly known and dreaded illnesses as pneumonia or the venereal diseases responded rapidly and positively to treatment. Previous therapy had been long, arduous, and possibly ineffectual. Interestingly, the frequent inclusion of a qualifying term, such as ". . . because I have a sore throat," in the penicillin shot request probably expresses concern for status. The qualification may be felt to preclude the possibility of a morally stigmatizing venereal disease. At any rate, penicillin cured rapidly—one of the miraculous aspects.

That penicillin was publicized as a miracle drug was extremely significant in the religiously oriented South. Association of the word "miracle" need not be elaborated, but the positive value related to religion does need stressing in this context. If they were miraculous, the penicillin shots were doubly good.

For patients, the shots had an aura of science, and scientific progress also had assumed general positive value, even in rural areas, where technological changes were attributed to science. The general lack of knowledge was still another facet of the miraculous aspect. That which is good and is mysterious often may be seen as miraculous. There was the sterilization ritual for both the needle and the skin. An intricate procedure involved filling the syringe as, almost ceremoniously, it was held up to the light and the contents were carefully measured—usually in the patient's presence. It all seemed very scientific!

Besides, the shots hurt; and in the South, if not elsewhere, everyone knew that "good medicine" is strong and tastes bad and, by analogy, if it hurt, it must be good. Also, the medicine was "put in" the body and could "go right to work," thus coinciding nicely with the mechanistic orientation. After the first generation, and then their children, had been so treated, there was the additional element of veneration by time. Shots became tried and true, because Papa and Mama vouched for them. Finally, the patient need not involve himself in this treatment. "Taking the medicine" occurred at the doctor's office, thus removing a patient's responsibility for accurate doses at proper times. It may be noted that this facet of the process also recommends "shots" to the physician—he can be sure his treatment modality has been effected. The efficacy of penicillin was established even further in rural areas, because it was used successfully with livestock—usually by injection.

A final aspect of the information lag pertains to physicians practicing in rural areas. For many of these men, the advent of antibiotics occurred during their educational years. They had been trained to see these treatment modalities as the most up-to-date and most effective. Practices that have become habitual are difficult to discard, particularly when such practices fit appropriately with long, harassing work days. This is not to malign the many physicians who most conscientiously keep apace of current academic developments. Patients with whom physicians have long-established, good relationships, however, obviously feel strongly about penicillin shots. Therefore, certain physicians may feel it advisable to maintain the cooperative relationship, thus facilitating continuing care delivery. An alienated patient could feel sufficiently rejected to refuse to accept *any* medical attention, no matter how badly needed. The relevant point is that it has continued to be possible for patients to receive shots of penicillin or of some placebo they believe to be penicillin.

Because the empirical experiences tended to retain positive value over time and were consistent within cultural values, there were varying degrees of internal reinforcement among the experiences. Here too, the other reinforcing elements are the relative insularity, the comparatively lower education level, and the introspective world view of the rural community.

A further consideration in this analysis concerns the place of ideal sex roles in the pattern. Rural southern ideal sex roles continue to be relatively differentiated. In illness behavior, role expression requires the male to be strong, stalwart, and able to "go 'til he can't go no more." He seeks medical treatment only when he is considered to be verging on collapse—in a crisis state. On the other hand, the female role includes acknowledgment of long-term frailty or suffering; she is expected to be "puny" and "ailing" and even "faintified." Her seeking medical care is legitimized at any time. Denial of penicillin injections produces anger, because it signals "you are not sick." To the male, this means he is "not much of a man," else he would not be seeking medical attention in the first place. To the female, it means negation of a portion of her whole orientation as a woman. To be given a penicillin shot is absolute evidence of illness, further enhancing its position of value in the belief system.

The analysis supports the thesis that the attitude involved in the penicillin shot syndrome can be considered a contemporary folk belief. There has been persistence over time, in that, in certain cases, it is now into the third generation. That the belief draws on a common pool of empirical experience was demonstrated. Because the belief is deeply rooted and consistently reinforced through the southern value system, it seems safe to predict that it will enjoy even further longevity. To date, its only known opposition would be an effective, universal educational program, combined with reduced instances of positive experiences.

A final contemporary note concerning folk beliefs and practices is appropriate. The current trend, particularly among the youth, toward "natural living," health foods, organic gardening, and the like, has produced a renaissance in folklore. Many older volumes of traditional beliefs and practices are reappearing in book stores and are being diligently studied and faithfully used. The movement also involves relocating in more rural settings, with gradual impetus toward the most remote areas. As interactions between the "newcomers" and the "oldtimers" become established, one can envision a further cross-reinforcement of folk beliefs and practices in rural areas.

SUMMARY

This discussion places folk understandings, beliefs, and practices in the cultural context of the people of Lafayette County. Folk beliefs are part of the self-treatment behavior patterns, which may be conceptualized as ranging along a continuum. This continuum moves from magic, at one end, to verbal formulas to remedies using plants and household materials through patent medicine and TV medicine to the currently emerging contemporary folk beliefs at the other end.

Further, this discussion sheds light on the dynamics involved in the developmental process concerning folk beliefs. The process seems to require the following elements. Positive empirical experiences must be fed into a common pool of knowledge. The experiences and consequent belief must be consistent with, and confirmed by, the group's value system. There must be multiple reinforcement over a period of time, preferably from some of the major institutions of the society and compatible with the social organization. Several characteristics of folk beliefs were presented and illustrated. These characteristics include a dynamic quality, tenacity, transportability, adaptability, and cultural expressivity.

In conclusion, this examination of the dynamics of rural folk belief, both traditional and modern, has served several functions. It provided an opportunity to consider the developmental process of folk tradition. It demonstrated that folk beliefs do not pertain exclusively to exotic or ancient peoples but are part of contemporary life-styles in the United States. The research method and analytic format could be applied in any setting to other behavior patterns. Specifically, it should be valuable knowledge, whereby health care deliverers may better understand extant beliefs and concomitant behavior. Thus, health education may be more effectively taught and health care more efficiently delivered.

IX. Doctor-Patient Communication in the Black Community of a Rural County

Margaret B. DiCanio, Ph.D.

THE FOLLOWING INCIDENT illustrates the type of inadequacy that may exist in communication in medical transactions; it also emphasizes the need for research aimed at improving such communication.

Standing in a supermarket checkout line, an elderly black lady began a conversation with this researcher. She told of her visit earlier that morning with the doctor at a public health clinic. She said the doctor had instructed her to get a board for her bed. Nodding, the researcher said politely in return, "Oh, you must be having trouble with your back." She agreed. Cocking her head to one side questioningly, she said, "Does the board have to be a new one, or reckon can I get a second-hand one over to the lumber yard?" The researcher explained that the quality the doctor had in mind was not newness, but flatness so she would not sleep with her back crooked. Whereupon the lady replied, "Oh—it doesn't go under the bed, it goes under the mattress."

Eight years of experience in three different paramedical fields reinforced the awareness of doctor-patient communication difficulties and created an impression that patients often emerged from interviews with physicians manifesting symptoms of uneasiness. Their anxiety seemed to center upon whether they had told the doctor all of their important symptoms and, if they had not, whether the omission would critically affect the course of treatment they were expected to follow. Perhaps because of their disquietude, often they were anxious also about whether they could remember the treatment procedure instructions.[1]

THE SETTING AND ITS PEOPLE

The presence of the newly opened teaching clinic in Lafayette County and the existence of the nearby black community provided the opportunity to explore systematically the above impression. With the exception of, at most, twenty individuals, the entire black population of the county (approximately 10 percent of the total 2,889) lives within relatively easy walking distance of the clinic. The Quarters are tucked away out of sight in a copse of trees. Although physically it is only a short distance from the downtown area, it gave the impression of isolation as the flatwoods push against one of its perimeters. It has one paved road. The other roads are collections of potholes that become quagmires or dust bowls, depending upon the weather.

Trying to find patients provided a number of "rural-urban cultural shocks." A post-office box number, or "general delivery," does not fix an address in space as concretely as does a named street and a house with a number. Directions, courteously given, came replete with assumptions acquired by years of living in the same locality. A small set of surnames with a high level of popularity made it problematic on many occasions as to whether the interviewer had connected with the correct patient household. To cope with the difficulties of finding the correct patient household, as well as for a control of nonpatient households, the researcher finally decided to visit all seventy-six of the Quarters' households. Among the total population, patient households were to be designated as those in which some member had been to the clinic by the time the interview was conducted. Conversely, households from which no member had visited the clinic were designated "nonpatient households."

In the black community there were four churches and one general store. These were among the best constructed buildings in this area. Twenty-four percent of the houses were owned by the occupants, almost half of which were trailers—for the most part, the best

1. The material in this chapter is from DiCanio, 1971.

existing housing. Housing was arbitrarily classified on a five-point scale from "good" to "hazardous." The "hazardous" housing, about 25 percent of the occupied dwellings, was only slightly better than being outdoors. Another 29 percent was beyond repair, although not necessarily hazardous to the health of the occupants.

Forty-one percent of the households had outdoor plumbing and three houses lacked even outhouses. (Subsequent to this study and as a result of combined efforts of a member of the clinic staff and the county sanitarian, new privies were provided for all houses, as needed.) Three houses had no electricity and used kerosene lamps. Several houses had diminutive wood-burning stoves that warmed only the side of the body turned toward them. They crackled threateningly amidst the dried old wood of the houses and were a source of peril for unsteady toddlers who ventured near.

At the time of this study, there was a school, constructed during the 1950s, for grades one through eight situated on one perimeter of the Quarters. This facility was closed when the county school system became totally integrated in 1969, and it is currently unoccupied.

During the 7-month study period, 142 individual patients from the black community visited the clinic for a total of 285 visits. Sixty-eight of the individuals were under age fifteen, but they accounted for only 85 visits. Thus, although half of the black patients were children, they accounted for only one-third of the visits. The children probably served as an introduction to the clinic for the whole household. This introduction may have resulted from the "sick-call" then being held every morning by the clinic staff at the district school. Notes were sent home to parents when medical care was thought advisable.

Prior to this "educational event," school activities apparently had not had a great deal of impact upon the daily lives of district residents. Surprisingly, though, 42 percent of the entire group had had a grade school education or better. Some of the older residents were careful to explain that in "their time" school only lasted a few months of the year and often cost "a dollar a head."

The attainment of a high school diploma did not seem to deter graduates from working in the tobacco fields along with those who had never been to school. Occupations of Quarters residents fell into unskilled categories, with a few exceptions that might be called semiskilled. The largest single categories involved work with the timber industry or in the tobacco fields of local growers. Most of the available work was seasonal, subject to weather fluctuations, and without any fringe benefits. Among those no longer able to work were some who described themselves as "too old and wore out to work" or as having been hurt on the job in timbering enterprises long since having moved on.

Obviously, both occupation and housing choices have been limited for Quarters residents. Until the advent of the clinic, health care choices had been equally limited. The nearest medical care had been twenty-five miles in one direction and twenty-seven miles in another. For those without a car, the only way to reach medical care was to have someone drive them, for a fee of five dollars. Even with the payment of the transportation fee, the choice of physician often depended upon the direction in which the driver was headed.

The distances to physician services effectively precluded pre-natal care. Midwives are coming back in style in modern medicine, but for the Quarters they have only recently gone out of style. Midwife deliveries accounted for 82 percent of the babies born to mothers in nonpatient households and 61 percent born to mothers in patient households.

The retirement of the local doctor and of the two midwives, together with the younger age of the patient households, probably explains why 31 percent of their babies were hospital deliveries in contrast to only 15 percent of the nonpatient households. The apparent increase in hospitalization is probably not as much a matter of increased awareness of the value of hospitalization as it is a reduction in the available alternatives. The implementation of a federally funded Mother-Infant Care program for high-risk patients within a hundred-mile radius of Shands Teaching Hospital also improved maternity hospitalization rates.

There is no intention of implying a lack of awareness about the need for good medical care on the part of the Quarters' residents but rather a difference in the ordering of priorities between the rural layman's realities and the medical profession's realities. Any suspicion about such a lack of awareness on the part of this rural community tended to be dispelled by this study.

An accumulation of casual comments in connection with the study indicated an attitude that is probably common even beyond the boundaries of this community. Some individuals who had had a previously diagnosed and treated illness were, upon its recurrence, less likely to return to the doctor on the grounds that they already knew what the illness was. A frequent question and answer pattern was something like this: "Would you go to a doctor if you had _____ ?" "If I never had it before, I would." This sounded reasonable until a respondent said this in connection with her "high blood." She had a prescription for her hypertension which had been depleted two years previously and never renewed.

RESEARCH DESIGN AND RESULTS

With the intent of examining the previously mentioned impression of patients' uneasiness following interactions with physicians, patients from the Quarters were interviewed in their homes shortly after their visits with the clinic's student-physicians. The purpose was to see whether the patient felt he had been given sufficient time to tell the doctor everything he wanted to tell him, whether the patient felt that the doctor had understood him, whether the patient had understood the doctor, and whether the patient could repeat what had transpired during his transaction with the doctor.

To get at the doctor's half of the transaction, it was decided to examine the medical record rather than interview the doctor. This choice was based on three factors: several interviews might be required of any one student-physician, thus skewing the response to the interview; the rotation of medical staff precluded assured availability of specific students; there was a possibility that interviewing might alter the behavior of student-physicians in patient transactions, thus making them less representative. In addition, the medical record prepared by a student-physician is probably among the better medical records, because he prepares it anticipating review by his instructors.

The choice of the black patients was to provide whatever measure of homogeneity possible for the patient population contraposed to the student-physician population. Also, the entire black community had not previously been involved in any studies carried out in the county.

Reasoning that residents of the Quarters who sought medical care might be different in some respects from those who did not, a symptom list developed by Koos was chosen to be administered to members of the community who had been treated at the clinic and to a central group who had not sought medical services from the clinic. The list contains seventeen symptoms, all of which require medical treatment. Each respondent was asked whether he would seek medical care for each of the seventeen symptoms. Koos had found that lower-class respondents viewed symptoms as being less serious than did respondents from higher socioeconomic levels.

The demands of the Quarters' rural dialect required substituting appropriate synonyms for some items of the Koos list and prompted using a semifocused interview in preference to a structured questionnaire. A tape recorder was used to keep the interview flexible and relaxed. It was promised at the outset that the tape would be erased in his presence, if the interview caused the respondent any discomfort. Once set up, the tape recorder was ignored and caused few problems.

The interviews lasted twenty to forty minutes, during which the Koos list was administered, questions about the clinic and clinic visits were asked, demographic data were gathered, and information about previous health care was elicited. Data were gathered to include all members of the household, to whatever level the interviewee could provide. School and clinic records helped to fill in some of the gaps. Residents were not voluble; on the other hand, they were not aloof. They seemed to enjoy being interviewed.

The oldest man in the community (aged 99) provided the only incomplete interview. He answered every question with a question. He had so much fun, though, that four of his neighbors were sufficiently reassured by watching that they sat one-by-one on his porch to be interviewed on that same afternoon.

Koos had found in Regionville that recognition of need for medical care increased with rising socioeconomic level. The Quarters patient and nonpatient groups differ in their recognition, although there was no apparent difference in their socioeconomic level. Recognition in the Quarters patient group seemed to fall between Koos' upper classes (I and II), and the Quarters nonpatients seemed to fit between Koos' lower classes (II and III). Granted, it is hardly remarkable that patients define symptoms as more serious than do nonpatients. This research suggests that there are intraclass distinctions, however, while Koos' work made the distinction between classes (see Table 1).

A possibility anticipated by the interviewer was that the Quarters residents' limited language skills would cause communication problems in the doctor-patient transaction. A possibility only dimly perceived was that this skill level would create problems for the interviewer in trying to obtain sufficient information about what had taken place in the medical transaction.

TABLE 1

PERCENTAGE OF REGIONVILLE'S THREE CLASSES
AND OF PATIENTS AND NONPATIENTS FROM THE QUARTERS
WHO RECOGNIZE SYMPTOMS AS REQUIRING MEDICAL ATTENTION

| | Regionville, Classes | | | The Quarters | |
	I	II	III	Patients	Nonpatients
Loss of appetite	57	50	20	64	52
Persistent backache	53	44	19	76	65
Continued coughing	77	78	23	82	60
Persistent joint and muscle pains	80	47	19	63	48
Blood in stool	98	89	60	87	73
Blood in urine	100	93	69	94	73
Excessive vaginal bleeding	92	83	54	75	66
Swelling of ankles	77	76	23	72	60
Loss of weight	80	51	21	59	44
Bleeding gums	79	51	20	45	30
Chronic fatigue	80	53	19	65	22
Shortness of breath	77	55	21	90	74
Persistent headaches	80	56	22	77	52
Fainting spells	80	51	33	88	70
Pain in chest	80	51	31	88	74
Lump in breast	94	71	44	92	88
Lump in abdomen	92	65	34	100	84
	(N = 51)	(N = 335)	(N = 128)	(N = 47)	(N = 23)

Essentially the patient's version of the transaction was obtained by asking the following seven questions:

1. What was wrong? What made you go to the doctor?
2. What did you tell him?
3. Did he seem to understand you?
4. Did you understand him?
5. What did he say? What was wrong?
6. What did he tell you to do?
7. Do you remember how often you had to take the medicine?

Questions 3 and 4 were usually interpreted as criticism of the doctor and elicited a prompt defense. Characteristically, the patient, fist on hip and head nodding in punctuation, would say, "He examined me real good! He was real nice!"

In order to compare the two sides of the doctor-patient transaction, a five-category coding form was developed. The patient's version was transferred from the tapes and placed side by side with the extracted notes from the medical record. The two versions were then coded as matched or unmatched onto the coding form.

To cope with the dilemma of the patient's brevity, any information given elsewhere in the interview with the researcher was included in coding his version of the interview. The reasoning was that the interest was not in whether he could neatly answer the researcher's questions but in whether he came away from the doctor-patient transaction informed. Patients often presented additional information while they were responding to the seventeen-symptom list. The taped interview proved invaluable in this respect. A much more detailed presentation of the research methodology and validity may be found elsewhere.[2]

Since the major thrust of this study concerned communication, the previous research efforts of Smith, Bernstein, and Shaw and of Costanzo provided a useful framework. The assumptions that emerged were as follows:

1. The patient population uses a language that has been called a restricted code. Their code arises from years of living in the same community, sharing similar experiences involving kinship ties, similar educational exposure, and occupational opportunities. Theirs is a relatively unchanging world—a familiar one. The language needed to function in this setting has limited requirements for flexibility designed to meet the unknown or unexpected. Verbal elaborations are superfluous.
2. The doctor population also uses a restricted language code. Theirs is the result of vigorous training. The learning includes the acquisition of professional "jargon" and a shared body of assumptions.
3. Each of the participants in any conversational transaction comes into the transaction with assumptions and a coding style acceptable to his significant reference group. From these he defines a situation new to him.
4. In an ambiguous or unstructured situation, an individual is forced to use his own internalized standards as an anchor. The more ambiguous the situation, the less his willingness to accept items new or contrary to his frame of reference. The patient, in a

2. See DiCanio, 1971.

doctor-patient transaction, is in a situation vastly more ambiguous for him than for the doctor, since he has had little prior training or experience to prepare him.

5. The doctor has available to him, in addition to his restricted code, an elaborated code. He has acquired this elaborated code by living in nonhomogeneous situations, where encounters contain unpredictable qualities. The doctor usually shares this in common with the middle class and with urbanites who comprise the large portion of his patient constituency.

If the assumption is accepted that each participant comes into the medical transaction from a different coding population, it can then be assumed that communication will be less than perfect, if not difficult. The focus then falls on who will be more skillful in the use of language necessary to conduct a doctor-patient transaction. Since the doctor has two codes available to him, it seems reasonable to expect that in any doctor-patient transaction, the doctor will have an advantage and also the responsibility for ensuring meaningful communication. It follows that any patient will be at a disadvantage, whether he is a middle-class urbanite, using an elaborated code like the doctor's elaborated code, or a lower-class ruralite, using a restricted, community-oriented code.

Without getting into a discussion of the values involved in whether one participant or the other should come away better informed, it seems safe to assume that the doctor will emerge from the transaction better informed. In this study, his better informed status will be evident in a greater number of unmatched responses. If communication were perfect, all responses would be matched. Table 2 shows the distribution of doctors' and patients' responses.

Little actual misunderstanding was revealed by the findings of this study. There were only 7 contradictory matches for a total of 14 responses out of 634. Instead, a lack of consensus emerged. Almost half of the responses, 49 percent, were unmatched or unacknowledged by the co-participant. It cannot be said that the co-participant did not know the matching response; it can only be said that it was not sufficiently important to him to reproduce. (In the case of doctors and medical students, this meant that portions of the patient responses were not included in the medical record.)

Eighty-two percent of the total unmatched responses belonged to the doctors in that patients could not recall information included in the patient records. There is also no proof that all the information recorded by the doctor was communicated to the patient. This is consistent with others' findings (Ley and Spelman, 1967), in which only one-quarter of a group of outpatients was able to recall everything they had been told by the doctor, and almost half of this total-recall group had been told only two things.

TABLE 2

DISTRIBUTION OF DOCTORS' AND PATIENTS' RESPONSE
TOTALS WITHIN TRANSACTION CATEGORIES

Transaction Category	Doctors' Unmatched	Doctors' Matched	Patients' Matched	Patients' Unmatched	Totals
History	19	9	9	7	44
Symptoms	160	69[a]	69[a]	34	332
Diagnosis	21	19[b]	19[b]	3	62
In-clinic treatment	19	41[c]	41[c]	6	107
Home care treatment	19	10[d]	10[d]	6	45
Follow-up	13	19	19	2	53
TOTALS	251	167	167	58	643

[a] Includes 3 contradictions and 1 ambiguity.
[b] Includes 1 ambiguity.
[c] Includes 3 contradictions and 1 ambiguity.
[d] Includes 2 ambiguities.

Even when the doctors made an effort to see that their patients were informed, patients remained dissatisfied with communication (Ley and Spelman). Suggested causes for dissatisfaction are difficulties in understanding and remembering what was said. The Quarters' patients, however, were not dissatisfied with their communication. Yet 59 percent of the items the doctor considered important enough to include in the medical record were unrecalled by the patient. What have been referred to as difficulties in understanding and remembering were viewed in this study as a difference in the language coding norms of the group of significance to the coder. The concept of coding was emphasized to underscore the normative language behaviors that permit lack of communication to go undetected because of the unacknowledged assumptions in exchanges.

Others have suggested that improvement in following doctors' instructions could be effected by having patients write instructions down, thereby providing them with a record they can subsequently follow (Ley and Spelman). This deserves attention and further research, with the following qualifications. The patient's hidden assumptions must be ferreted out to assure that he understands the instruction. A means would have to be found to prevent the extension of time that the doctor spends with the patient. Otherwise doctors, who already feel burdened, would be unwilling to consider the method. It must be recognized that not all patients are literate or physically capable of writing.

Perhaps more effective than writing instructions would be to include in the medical team a member whose responsibility is translating from the medical code to the patient's and, then, follow-up. Taping or videotaping of doctor-patient transactions and follow-up interviews have been suggested elsewhere (Grotjahn, 1970). This could provide instruction reinforcement by playing tapes back for patients. It would also make available training material for medical personnel, and research data in communication transactions and doctor-patient communication in particular. (This would, of course, require special equipment and extra space, and at present would make the cost of the doctor-patient interaction prohibitive.)

The reading of eight or nine hundred medical records revealed some interesting behavior patterns. As conscientious as they are, student-doctors do not always read the patient's previous record. Procedures get ordered more than once, or previously ordered procedures are not carried out on subsequent visits. Conversion to the problem-oriented medical record system should help in alleviation of such difficulties. Efforts are being made to effect that record system conversion in the clinic.

Patients are often told that it is critical for them to return. When they do not, the record ends abruptly. Sometimes the student nurses contact the patients. In this respect, student medical practice at the Lafayette Health Center may deviate from the norm of general medical practice.

In general practice, when a doctor has had his say and the patient leaves the scene, the transaction may be ended. Yet this is contrary to scientific method, because outcomes are assumed before evidence is in. It is assumed that the patient will follow advice, and also that if he does not return, he must have regained his health; it is also possible, however, that he might have died or gone to another physician. Both patient and doctor suffer from not having their assumptions followed up and examined. The research suggests that some assumptions about the insularity of rural communities will need re-evaluation as the progress of television sets precedes the progress of plumbing. Television has informed viewers well about lumps in the breast being a sign of cancer, and about the benefits of Geritol® for "tired blood." Television also may account, to some extent, for the intraclass differences found in response to the Koos symptom list, discussed earlier.

The major health problems in the black community seemed to be inadequate housing and "outhousing," parasites, and extreme dental care needs. Unfortunately television can do little to change the environmental and socioeconomic conditions involved in these health problems. Nor could television have done much to change the locale of the delivery of babies. This research revealed that 63 percent of the babies born to the residents of the Quarters were nonhospital deliveries. This is apparently a changing pattern as suggested earlier. The advent of the clinic will probably accelerate this and other changes.

EXPLANATORY STATEMENT

The project reported was conducted during the first year of the clinic's operation. It provided results in two general areas: a systematic examination of doctor-patient communication within the black community of Lafayette County and a sophisticated technique for recording, coding, and analyzing statistical research data. Also, it provided an objective description of the black community in Lafayette County. In keeping with the theme of this book, primary emphasis was given to the material related to the health needs and care of the residents of Lafayette County. Interest in the second general area may be satisfied by means of its publication elsewhere (DiCanio, 1971).

A brief comment concerning utilization of the teaching clinic by the black population of Lafayette County seems appropriate. On the first day of operation, no blacks attended and the staff expressed interest in the possible cause. Two or three blacks presented on the second day, and, by the end of the first week as well as thereafter, attendance at the clinic by blacks accurately reflected the black-white ratio of the population.

Professional Education and
Rural Health

FROM ITS INCEPTION, the Lafayette County Health Center has provided educational as well as service and research functions. In this section, faculty members centrally involved in establishing medical and nursing education programs based in this rural clinic discuss the problems and promise of these endeavors.

The chapter on medical education is about the impact of emerging community medical education programs upon traditional hospital-oriented teaching. It contains the development of a university-related rural program, indicating the unique advantages and difficulties posed by such a teaching setting. Concrete incidents are given, illustrating specific kinds of learning effectively offered in the rural health care setting. The chapter is concluded with consideration of the implications of this model for broader use in medical education.

The second chapter moves from a consideration of the nature of community nursing to examination of the effect of the rural setting on nursing practice and the advantages offered by a rural health center for nursing education programs. The description of the program in Lafayette County is illuminated by anecdotes and quotations from students. The impact of these learning experiences on the students' relationships with other health professionals and with patients is discussed.

X. Medical Education in a Rural County

Leighton E. Cluff, M.D.

AT THE BEGINNING of this century, Flexner, Welch, Osler, and other visionaries of medical education emphasized the importance of the teaching hospital as the "laboratory of the clinical teacher." Their influence led medical schools to develop their own teaching hospital or hospitals as the principal, if not only, location for training of physicians. This resulted in extraordinary advances in understanding of disease, development of sophisticated medical technology, enhancement of scholarship, improvements of hospital patient care, and enlargement of the scientific base of medical practice. It would be foolhardy to overlook these accomplishments or to retard their further development. As these events have evolved, however, the character of many teaching hospitals has changed, resulting in their becoming centers for the care of patients with complicated, complex, and serious illnesses, requiring the attention of highly trained personnel and specialized facilities. Associated with these changes, many teaching hospitals are less often used for primary or comprehensive patient care (if they ever were). This shapes the interest, perspective, and qualifications of faculty and physicians in training. No one could rightly question the importance of sustaining the teaching hospitals as they are essential if new accomplishments are to be fostered in the future. Whether they should continue to be the primary or only location for medical education, however, is in doubt.

Hospitalized patients are a small portion of those needing medical care, and the proportion of patients cared for in teaching hospitals

141

is even smaller. The majority of persons requiring medical care are not hospitalized. Emphasis upon training of physicians in teaching hospitals, therefore, is narrowly focused. Inculcation of interest, perspective, and qualifications of physicians in wider aspects of medical care require development of additional educational opportunities elsewhere.

The recent attention given to educational programs in community health and family medicine reflects awareness by the public and the medical profession of the need for training opportunities to be added to those available in the university medical center and hospital. The community educational programs developed must take advantage of the opportunity available locally. Programs in large urban centers may differ from those in rural areas, but they should have similar objectives.

The objectives and purposes of community medical training programs are several; some are similar to those in the teaching hospital, others are different. The emphasis, however, is more patient or people oriented than disease oriented. The opportunity for detection, investigation, and understanding of disease in the community, however, must be recognized and fostered.

ONE COMMUNITY MEDICAL EDUCATION PROGRAM

The University of Florida College of Medicine is located in north central Florida. Its teaching hospital serves as a referral center for a large area in which two or more million persons live. The hospital and its clinics do not usually serve as a primary or secondary facility for care of patients in the City of Gainesville or Alachua County, the site of the Medical School and University Hospital. The surrounding area is largely rural, and a few counties have had no doctor for ten or more years. The people in these counties, therefore, have had to seek their medical care thirty or more miles from their homes.

From 1966 to 1968, a medical center committee, appointed by the vice president for health affairs, discussed the proposals and plans of different departments for development of community educational and patient-care programs. Over a year much was said but nothing was done, illustrating the difficulty in evolving an institution-wide thrust in this field.

Discussions were begun in 1966 at residents' morning report in the Department of Medicine to evaluate the house staff 's interest in participating in and developing a community health care program in which they would assume important responsibilities. Encouraged by their responsiveness and enthusiasm, several surrounding communities were visited to determine their suitability as sites for a clinic. It became clear, however, that a community educational program must provide continuity of patient care and this could be assured only by enlisting a member of the faculty to devote his time to its development. Discussion with several members of the faculty in 1966–67 demonstrated lukewarm interest and antagonism to the project. For them it often represented a diversion of time and resources to an activity not in their academic interest. A decision had to be made to proceed without significant faculty support or to abandon the effort. Fortunately, the vice president for health affairs was encouraging and gave his moral, but no financial, support to the undertaking.

Discussions with a former colleague, who had been practicing general internal medicine in a small rural community in Maryland for nine years but had maintained an active part-time academic involvement at the Johns Hopkins Medical School, provided insight into the approaches required and problems to be met in development of a community medical education program. Solicitation of his counsel kindled his interest, and he agreed to accept an appointment to the faculty of the Department of Medicine to evolve a community medical program, with the initial emphasis upon providing opportunities for residents in internal medicine to obtain perspective of the medical care needs and the role of the physician in the community.

Limited resources of the Department of Medicine were allocated for planning and early development of a community program. Initially, the person recruited to initiate the project was also given responsibility for the Teaching Hospital's General Medical Clinic, and served, like other members of the faculty, as an attending physician to the inpatient medical service. This proved to be important as it enabled him to sustain his strong clinical abilities and established his position as an academician and teacher. It was understood from the beginning that the ambulatory and community-based programs must include investigative activities to allow them to compete effectively in the academic setting and to meet their academic opportunities and responsibilities. The subsequent growth and development of the program indicate the importance of this earlier assumption. A Division of Ambulatory Care and Community Programs was established to provide recognition for the project and to facilitate involvement of the chief of the program in deliberations by the Departmental Executive Committee. These efforts have been important in establishing the program as an academic unit and have kept it involved in department and college planning. In addition, it has provided a means for informing and involving other faculty members and programs in its activities.

In the beginning, visits were made to several patient care and medical educational programs throughout the country to gain familiarity with other programs under development elsewhere. The rural area of north Florida was visited to become familiar with the needs, interest, and settings available for development of a clinical program. Several objectives were identified to meet our academic aims and resources: the area should be medically deprived; the population to be served should not exceed five thousand to avoid a patient-care load which might limit its use as an educational unit; the community leaders should be enthusiastic about development of a patient care and educational program for which they and the Medical School would be responsible; the location should be sufficiently distant (in excess of 25 miles) from the Health Center to necessitate residence of house staff in the community rather than enabling the house staff and students to commute each day to the clinic from their homes in Gainesville.

Several counties proved suitable for the program. Lafayette County, with the county seat, Mayo, sixty miles from Gainesville, was seen as most satisfactory. It had a new clinic building occupied only by an itinerant sanitation officer serving another county and by a public health nurse, who had the major responsibility for providing health care in the county. The community leaders were enthusiastic about the possible establishment of a medical care and educational program in their clinic building and were eager to assist in development and supervision of the program. A Citizens' Advisory Committee with minority group (black) representation was established and served as the mechanism for implementation of the program.

The dean of the College of Medicine was advised of our efforts and intentions but expressed concern about reaction of the physicians in the state to inauguration of such a community program. This hastily precipitated a meeting with the chairman of the University President's Medical Advisory Committee, a distinguished internist residing some one hundred miles from the College of Medicine. He cautiously supported our undertaking, when he was convinced that our primary objective was to develop an important new educational opportunity and not only to expand into a new patient-care program. The State Medical Society finally supported the program and formed a committee of physicians to oversee its development.

In January 1968, the clinic was opened by a second-year medical resident, who moved his family to Mayo, Florida, for two months, and since then, the medical residents have been rotated through the clinic at monthly intervals. Three senior medical students, relieved of their duties in the General Medical Clinic of the University Hospital, joined the assistant resident. Subsequently, three to five senior students were rotated through the clinic at three-week intervals during their nine-week required involvement in the Department of Medicine's Medical Clinic Program. Housing for the resident and his family was provided by renting a house in the town, and the students initially lived in the only motel in town but now live in a mobile home adjacent to the clinic. The faculty member recruited to develop and oversee the program, one other faculty member, and the Department of Medicine chairman provided regular supervision of the patient care program and developed an educational basis for the resident physician and students during the first eighteen months; now other faculty are involved as well. The department chairman held professorial rounds in the clinic every Wednesday morning at which clinical, medicosocial, and medicoeconomic questions or problems identified by the students or residents were discussed.

An early concern was the viability of the clinic program after our first blush of enthusiasm. The rotation of residents in medicine through the clinic as part of their required experience, and the rotation of students at three-week intervals, in addition to the support of the chief of the Division of Ambulatory and Community Programs, chairman of the Department of Medicine, dean, a small number of the faculty, and the community have sustained the clinic now for over four years. The resident physician has been the key to the success of the program. He is there all of the time, even when students are on vacation and he is alone. At times a faculty member spells him briefly, particularly on holidays. His role is to oversee the patient-care program on a twenty-four-hour basis, teach the students, work with the community and nurses. Usually, his wife and children live with him in the community for one month, and this proves to be an important experience for them as well. Some of the wives have made significant contributions to the clinic or community.

The resident physician and students moving to the clinic for four or three weeks, respectively, have additional expenses during this time. They are obliged to maintain their housing in Gainesville, establish residence in Mayo, and have travel expenses to and from Mayo. The students and resident physician have been given per diem funds to cover their added expenses. Initially, this was covered by departmental resources but, subsequently, by College of Medicine funds and foundation grants. Income from patient care now pays the expenses of the resident physician, but otherwise educational costs have not been borne by patient fees.

Early on, all residents were interested in participating in the program, perhaps because of its novelty. Subsequently, some residents who have served in the Armed Forces as medical officers have felt the community clinic duplicates the military experience because the medical problems arising have been similar. The nonmedical aspects of the program, however, are not the same and provide a different perspective, for those able to see it. Rarely has a resident physician resisted openly his assignment to the clinic. On two occasions when this occurred, a prior visit to the clinic with the department chairman eliminated their resistance and in each instance these residents found the experiences valuable, retrospectively. If provided only as an elective to resident physicians probably only one-third or fewer would seek to work in the clinic. Nevertheless, over 80 percent of them attest to the value of the program after they have participated in it. Some residents view the month in Mayo as a relaxing break from their hospital responsibilities; others find the per diem payment above their usual stipend an incentive. Sharing of the experience by all residents has provided an esprit de corps among them, and often their individual experiences become the subject of discussion at social functions when they return to Gainesville. No resident has subsequently entered practice in a small rural community, but this was not the objective of the program. The hope was that they would have a better perspective of the health needs of the public and the physician's role in meeting these needs, enabling them to more reasonably meet and deal with these needs, wherever and however they functioned later on. A few residents have extended their training, following their residency, into fields related to the program, one to obtain an MPH degree in Health Care at Johns Hopkins University's School of Public Health and Hygiene; another has developed a primary interest in medical administration. Still another has assisted in establishment of health care delivery programs in surrounding areas while serving in the Armed Forces in another state. The ultimate influence of the program upon these residents in internal medicine must await further evaluation. It is likely that the existence of this community program has influenced some medical graduates to seek or avoid our house staff program in internal medicine, but during its existence the academic qualifications of the house staff have markedly improved, and the number applying for positions has risen markedly. Conceivably, some have applied because of the existence of the program.

Until one and one-half years ago, only senior medical students who had completed their required traditional clinical clerkships were involved in the community program. While working in the community clinic, they were on call twenty-four hours a day, were obliged to make house calls, and cared for patients in the clinic on a rotational basis, much as in the teaching hospital. With the development of a new educational program or curriculum for the students a few years ago, however, the community program was made a required part of the regular clinical clerkship. This was a recognition of the value of the program in medical education and was welcomed but presented a new problem and concern. Many of the faculty felt that students should not be involved in the community program, at least, until they had completed their required clerkship in medicine and pediatrics in the teaching hospital. This proved to be impossible logistically. Subsequently, however, the students assigned to the clinic in their sophomore and junior years have functioned well. The only qualification is that those students whose first or second clinical clerkship rotation is in the community clinic are more hesitant and insecure, and require greater supervision by the resident physician. After this, however, they function equally as well as senior students did before. At one point, both senior and junior students worked together in the clinic, and it was possible to compare their performances. This has reinforced our belief that students need not have completed their in-hospital clerkships to function well in a community program.

The importance of the community experience to the students is best illustrated by the description provided by one student at the conclusion of his involvement.

As an experience in medical education, the clinic offers several unique opportunities. The patient population is unselected, with the physical and emotional, the benign and the morbid, and the subclinical and the end-stage of disease thrown together. A knowledge of human behavior and culture is essential in order to function efficiently in such a setting. Skill is required in the practice of meeting the needs of the patient as the patient sees them and in being able to withstand the anxiety, both yours and the patient's, of not being able to call the patient's difficulty by name or arrive at a diagnosis. In day-to-day practice of medicine, this particular goal is achieved with clarity in only a small percentage of cases. It was fascinating to observe how the patient's concept of "good medical care" came to influence my approach to self-limited, generally benign processes.

Whether or not the medical students involved in this community program over the past few years have been influenced in identifying career choices remains to be seen. Nevertheless, it is likely that their attitudes toward medical care have been enlarged, and we hope they will be better prepared to provide leadership and provide better care for their patients later on.

Some students have been relieved of the responsibility of participating in the community program for personal reasons: a pregnant wife, etc. No student, however, has ever resisted participation in the clinic. The duration of the students' involvement in the clinic has been kept at three weeks. Less than this would be too short and longer than this might not be further productive.

Rotation of students and the resident physician at three and four weeks, respectively, usually makes it possible to provide overlapping involvement in the patient care program. In addition, each new resident overlaps the preceding resident by a day or two to facilitate smooth operation of the clinic.

Many experiences during the past four years provide insight into the value, importance, and reasons for existence, as well as evidence of problems in the program. Some of these will be described, anecdotally, for illustrative purposes. Many investigative and evaluative studies have been done but will not be presented here.

The Flu and Mumps Outbreak: The Role of the Physician in Public Education

Shortly after the clinic opened an influenza epidemic developed in the community (February 1968). The resident physician and medical students were overwhelmed with the increased number of patients coming to the clinic for care. The Department of Medicine chairman, during a regular Wednesday morning visit, discussed the management of this problem. Most of the patients needed only rest, fluids, and supportive care in the home. Few complications of influenza which required the physician's attention were recognized. Most patients or the parents of children with influenza were frightened, needed reassurance, and wanted guidance. The suggestion was made to prepare a "Health Message" for the local newspaper, which was read by most persons in the county, advising them as to what influenza is, what to do for the affected person at home, and when to seek medical attention. The students and the resident prepared this message, and it was published in the paper shortly thereafter. Within twenty-four hours, the frequency of visits to the clinic declined markedly, and those patients appearing usually required attention of the physician. This illustrated the importance of providing information to the public about health matters and demonstrated how this could influence the demands upon the physician's time and skill and the patient's ability to care for himself.

A similar event, with precisely the same sequence, occurred some months later when an outbreak of mumps developed in the community (see Chapter III).

This experience illustrated for the resident physician and medical students, as well as the faculty, the important role of the physician in health education. The students and residents in the clinic have since periodically published other health messages in the local newspaper. The impact of this upon the community is difficult to assess but certainly has improved use of the clinic for medical care.

Community Action and Worms

A few months after the opening of the clinic, one of the medical students recognized that several patients seen in the clinic, particularly children, had intestinal worms. She took it upon herself to determine what was known about the frequency of intestinal parasitism in the southeastern United States and found little new information developed in the past several years. She, therefore, did a sample survey of the children in the elementary school in the community and, with the assistance of the State Health Department Laboratory, characterized the nature of the intestinal parasitism in children in the community and identified the parasites responsible for infection. About 80 percent of the school children had some form of intestinal parasitism. The incidence appeared to be higher in those living in one section of the community, locally referred to as "the Quarters," composed mostly of black families. The Quarters were in a low-lying area, the soil was frequently wet, and there were inadequate sewage disposal facilities. Many of the homes had outdoor privies or there were no privies at all. It seemed likely that defecation was occurring away from the homes. The intestinal parasites responsible for infection included *Trichina*, hookworm, and roundworm or *Ascaris*.

At this time Dr. Henry Meleney, certainly one of the world's foremost parasitologists, was professor emeritus on the staff of the Department of Medicine. He became interested in the problem and consulted with the students and resident physician as to what might be done to eliminate the problem of intestinal parasitism in the community. Consideration was given to the possibility of mass treatment of the affected children. Dr. Meleney recognized, however, that this would be unlikely to control the problem permanently until the Quarters area had been cleaned up and privies and adequate drainage of the area had been provided. Dr. Meleney initiated efforts on the part of the medical students and the resident, contacting the local school principals and high school students, as well as the community leaders and, during a summer month, led this team to remove the debris and clean up the Quarters. He acquired outdoor privies for those houses which did not have indoor toilets and influenced the community leaders to plant trees in the area and drain the swampy ground. As a result of this effort, Dr. Meleney was recognized by the community and given an honorary award at the time of the high school graduation ceremonies. He presented appropriately labeled T-shirts to each of the contributing members of the high school, as well as to the medical students and resident involved in the clean-up campaign.

This type of experience, begun by a medical student, leading to an examination of an important health problem in the community, illustrates an important type of experience in community health education.

THE CHAIRMAN OF THE DEPARTMENT OF MEDICINE AS A STUDENT

When the clinic program had been in existence for about a year and a half, the chairman of the Department of Medicine decided he should function as a medical student in the clinic to gain a deeper appreciation of the problems, advantages, and other aspects of the medical student education program, as well as to have an opportunity to work with an assistant resident responsible for the patient-care program and the direction of the clinic activities.

During a two-week period when the medical students were on vacation, the chairman moved to Mayo to live in a mobile home which had been installed adjacent to the clinic for the medical students, and also took with him as a student the chairman of the Department of Microbiology. They functioned as medical students in the clinic for a two-week period. The assistant resident on the chairman's service at that time continued to function as the director and leader in the clinic, and the chairman of the Department of Medicine and the chairman of the Department of Microbiology cared for the patients coming to the clinic on a rotational basis as the medical students had done before. Some of the attitudes of the people living in the community toward the clinic became apparent as a result of that experience.

One morning a young boy was brought into the clinic by his mother. The young boy had an infected foot with lymphangitis and cellulitis, indicative of a streptococcal infection. The mother was advised by the chairman of the department of the nature of the boy's difficulty. The recommendation was made that treatment of the boy with penicillin would undoubtedly clear up the difficulty, but the mother indicated that she would appreciate it if the chief physician could see her boy before a final decision was made as to his disposition. This illustrated the awareness of people living in the community of the important role of the resident as the physician primarily responsible for the care program in the clinic. It also indicated that the age of the resident physician did not detract from his ability to assume this role, even though the chairman of the department was probably two times older than the assistant resident physician.

One Sunday, a telephone call to the clinic indicated that an elderly man previously seen for a cerebral vascular accident had become acutely ill. The chairman of the Department of Microbiology and the assistant resident physician, therefore, made a home visit, determined that the man had a urinary tract infection, possibly bacteremia, and required hospitalization. The chairman of the Department of Medicine, who was caring for the clinic while the others were making the home visit, was selected to escort the patient and his daughter into Gainesville by ambulance, serving as the ambulance driver as well as the physician. The hour drive into Gainesville and back provided an interesting and important type of experience which medical students may have while working in such a community.

The interest and support of the chairman of the Department of Medicine is critically important in stimulating enthusiasm and involvement of assistant residents and medical students in a community educational experience.

TOBACCO SICKNESS

After the clinic had been open for approximately two years, the assistant resident physician, one of the faculty, and the medical students became aware of a recurring problem during the harvesting of the tobacco crop. Many of the tobacco croppers developed rash, fever, nausea, and vomiting. The illness was well known to the residents of the community. A search of the literature revealed no previous reports of a similar problem. The residents of the community were interrogated, and it was found that the tobacco sickness had appeared each year during harvesting when the leaves were wet. The medical students attempted to relate this illness to the nicotine content of the tobacco leaf or the use of pesticides, and extracted tobacco leaf to identify the responsible agent. No definite results were obtained, but the description of a new illness was identified. This illustrates the opportunities in a community program for medical students to be involved in medical investigation. The physician in the community must have the ability to use epidemiological methods in providing medical care, and there is no better way for a medical student or a young physician in training to acquire this ability than in a community program.

DIGNITY IN DYING

One of the requirements of the medical students and the assistant resident in the clinic is to make house calls when necessary. The community has provided an automobile for this purpose. One particular instance illustrates the importance of home visits.

On one occasion, a woman called for assistance for her husband. The man had a high fever and was confused. A medical student, a student nurse, and the assistant resident physician visited the patient in his home. Upon entering the home, they met four sons of the sick patient and his wife. The sons had come home when they heard their father was ill. The patient was about 90. He had labored breathing, was coughing purulent sputum, had fever and evidence of pneumonia. He had been in bed for some time because of a stroke some years previously. The medical student and resident recommended that the patient be hospitalized. The family, however, requested that he be treated at home as he had been bedridden for some time, and they felt it important for their husband and father not to die away from home, fully recognizing the seriousness of his illness. With trepidation, the assistant resident physician and the medical student were impressed with the importance of the family's request and agreed. They administered penicillin to the patient and made frequent visits to the home to follow his course, but on the third day of illness he died. The family was grateful for the care that he had received and was appreciative of the concern and attention to their wishes.

This experience illustrates the importance of home visits in providing an experience for students and resident physicians in meeting the needs of patients under circumstances where considerations important to the patient and his family can be seen and appreciated.

THE SCHIZOPHRENIC PAPER BOY

As the assistant resident physician and the medical students live in the area, they become friendly with many of the residents of the community. On one occasion, the students and the resident physician discussed a middle-aged, schizophrenic man who sold newspapers each day in the center of town. He was brought to the clinic for evaluation of another problem, and it was recommended that he should be institutionalized for care. It became apparent, however, that the community was aware that the man was psychotic and had been for many years. The community had adapted to his problem, provided him with a job selling newspapers, and looked after him without institutionalization. The community did not want the patient institutionalized as they felt qualified in providing care for him themselves.

This illustrated for the students and the assistant resident physician that a community may be more qualified in caring for its chronically ill individuals than is a medical institution.

THE PUBLIC SCHOOLS

Teachers in the public schools have used the medical students, the assistant resident physician, and the student nurses in their educational programs. The medical students, assistant resident, and student nurses have conducted classes in the elementary school and the high school on dental hygiene, the health professions, venereal disease, and other health topics. An attempt was made to provide sex education for the students, but this was resisted by members of the community. The medical students and the assistant resident physician now are responsible for the physical examinations of the students entering the public schools within the county. This is sponsored by the local school board and is a regular responsibility of the clinic. Some of the local teachers have had the medical students dissect frogs and teach aspects of biology in their classes.

This illustrates another role of the physician in the community because of his knowledge of biology and health. These experiences have encouraged student nurses to conduct evening classes on first aid for the community, as farm injuries are common.

AN OUTBREAK OF DIPHTHERIA

Three years ago, a diphtheria outbreak occurred in Florida. There were a few deaths in south Florida, and several cases of diphtheria were recognized in a county adjoining Lafayette. The faculty, medical students, assistant resident physician, and student nurses, therefore, began a county-wide immunization program for diphtheria. Over a few days, almost all children in the county were immunized. This precipitated an interest in seeing that the county was adequately immunized against poliomyelitis, measles, pertussis, and tetanus. At the present time, the school children in the county are completely immunized against these diseases.

This illustrated for the students and resident the role of the physician in meeting the health needs of the population by development of regular immunization programs in the community.

MISCELLANEOUS

Many other experiences besides the ones cited demonstrate the importance of a community experience for medical students and physicians in training. It seems likely that the medical students and the assistant resident physicians of the Department of Medicine participating in this program over the past six years have a better familiarity with the health care needs of the public than any other similar group. They also probably have a better appreciation of the importance of the physician in the community in meeting the health needs of the public.

Before the clinic opened, a prepaid health care system was considered. The members of the Citizens' Advisory Committee, however, did not want a charity clinic, and they were not prepared to develop a prepaid system. They wanted a fee-for-service system. The Citizens' Advisory Committee, therefore, developed the fee system, and they are responsible, in part, for collecting these fees and overseeing the finances of the clinic. Funds have been allocated by the County Commission to meet some of the needs for the indigent population and to provide x-ray and other facilities for the clinic. Unfortunately, because of legal requirements, it was necessary to abandon the ambulance service. The cooperative relationship and shared responsibility for the clinic program by the medical staff and residents of the community must represent one of the few instances when medical care provided is not solely determined by the medical profession.

The appreciation of the population of the community for the clinic is illustrated in a number of ways. On one occasion, a local service station attendant indicated that he hoped he never had to use the clinic, but having the clinic in the community relieved his concern, because he now knew that when he got sick, he would not have to travel far to get assistance. The elimination of fear of illness in the community has been important.

The medical students, assistant resident physicians, and nursing students have been involved in the activities of the local churches and have been introduced by the ministers to members of the congregations. The assistant resident physician becomes an honorary member of the Rotary Club and attends weekly luncheon meetings where he comes to know more closely than otherwise possible some of the community leaders and learns of their concerns for the area in which they live.

Whether or not the clinic program has a prolonged effect upon the attitudes of the residents and the students remains to be determined. It seems likely, however, that it will have an impact upon their future professional activities.

It is important to note after six years that many of the faculty of the Department of Medicine and College of Medicine continue to view the community program as a diversion of resources of the institution into programs not in its best interests. This suggests that the development of such programs will not, for some time, achieve broad acceptance within the academic community. Nevertheless, this should not be a deterrent to the establishment of such programs.

The program described in Mayo, Florida, is only a beginning. Now that an experimental physicians' assistants program has been established in an adjoining county, the medical students, assistant resident physician, and nursing students have an opportunity to examine the role of the physician's assistant in the delivery of patient care. These physicians' assistants function in the Mayo clinic and some of the students have an opportunity to participate in their activities in the adjoining county. This provides a mechanism to evaluate the role of physicians' assistants in rural America.

Enlargement of the program is under consideration to develop other health care systems in nearby rural, medically deprived communities which could enhance the educational opportunities as well. Several other counties are deprived of medical care and could provide opportunities to develop enlarged comprehensive health care programs, serving as an enlarging base for medical education.

The program forcefully illustrates the dual role of a physician. His primary responsibility is care of individuals seeking his attention and services. His second, but also important, responsibility is to provide leadership in planning and implementing programs serving the population or all the people in the community. The traditional role of the physician in providing individual patient care is emphasized in the hospital and in the daily work of physicians. Involvement in community medical education programs, however, also emphasizes the role of the physician in meeting community health needs. Although this latter role has been taught in the past by courses in public health or preventive medicine, instruction in these areas has been disassociated from the role of the physician in caring for individuals. Only when these two responsibilities of the physician are integrated into a common or single educational program will it be possible for physicians in training to recognize their dual but mutually dependent roles.

XI. Nursing Education in a Rural County

June Remillet, R.N., M.A.

COMMUNITY HEALTH nursing practice began in New York City in 1877, sponsored by the Women's Board of the New York City Mission. District nurse associations were started in Boston and Philadelphia seven years later. Thus, historically the original delivery of community nursing services began and was concentrated in metropolitan areas by voluntary agencies. The rural population of the United States did not receive much attention from nursing until 1912, when the American Red Cross initiated a program named "Town and Country Nursing Service" in an effort to encourage each community to develop its own services, geared to local health and nursing needs. This program, which reached rural areas, was financed by contributions, fees, insurance company contracts, and sometimes community grants.

Outstanding and unusual for the time was Mary Breckinridge's "Nurses on Horseback," who gave prenatal care, midwife delivery, and postpartum follow-up in the remote rural areas of the mountains in Kentucky. This service was founded in 1925.

The W. K. Kellogg Foundation was established in 1930 to promote health education and the general welfare of mankind. One of the early projects of the foundation was the financing of local county health departments in southern Michigan, employing baccalaureate prepared nurses to work in the local rural health departments and to give a generalized service with emphasis on the health of children and expectant parents.

In 1934, the Division of Public Health Nursing (Florida) was created at the State Board of Health level through the Federal Emergency Relief Administration Nursing Project. Eleven supervisors and 275 county nurses were appointed to provide a generalized nursing program in public health with emphasis on maternal and child health, communicable disease control, and parent education.

During the first three decades of this century, rural community health programs were implemented sporadically. Though they were publicized to be generalized nursing programs, they tended to concentrate on the clinical areas mentioned, and in no way could they be called comprehensive health care for a given community. Simultaneously city health departments and voluntary visiting nurse associations were expanding and approaching better levels of care, where urbanization was feeling the impact of migration from the farmlands.

Various descriptions of public health nursing have much in common, though they stress different goals or purposes.

1. Dr. Ira Hiscock stated that "Public health nursing is a combination of bedside care of the ill and educational efforts to help others stay well."

2. Dr. John J. Hanlon paid particular attention to the service aspects of the public health nurse when he wrote, "It is people and families who are to be served by public health nurses rather than diseases or conditions."

3. Dr. Ruth B. Freeman wrote that public health nursing activities include "comprehensive nursing care of individuals, families, and groups, and, in addition, public health measures addressed to the community as a whole, such as epidemiologic investigations, law enforcement, or organization of the community for health action."

If the foregoing definitions encompass what community nursing is, and if the nurse is the core of the personal health service in a community, then community nursing is basically the same wherever the setting. The adaptations lie in the culture, the values, the economy, and the education of the population served. It is to these community-life aspects that the nurse must adapt her knowledge and skill. Philosophically the guidelines for service are not altered.

NURSING IN THE CONTEXT OF RURAL HEALTH CARE

When the majority of nursing students enrolled in a baccalaureate program are from middle-class families who have lived their entire lives in cities of 70,000 (population) or more, it is not likely they will find residing in a town of 700 people an equally stimulating environment. Not many graduate nurses prefer to live in the slow tempo of the rural village, unless it is their home or they originated from such a society. This may account, in part, for the sparsity of public health nurses in the rural portions of our country. It has been our favorable experience, however, to have more senior nursing students volunteer for the ten-week practicum with the Lafayette County Health Center than can be accommodated within the clinical area, the amount of clinical material, and the living quarters. Because this particular rural setting and the students' practicum are so vastly different from the relative protection of a large teaching hospital, it is gratifying to have students who volunteer to take their course work in this locale; one-fourth of the class competes for the available places.

Community health courses are offered through three quarters of the academic year. Four or five nursing students live, study, and learn in the Lafayette County Health Center each quarter. They are volunteers for this assignment. (Other students in the same courses have their laboratory elsewhere.) Students are screened during a private interview with an instructor. There are some criteria for judging the selectees:

1. The student must not have any dependents who would demand his / her absence from the laboratory, such as a child or spouse. In the case of the latter, if there is an understood agreement between the two, an exception might be made.
2. She / he must have safe transportation: car, motorcycle, etc.
3. If female, she must not be pregnant, because there are many miles of car travel required and many steps to be taken during a clinic session. For the protection of the student, the faculty believe she should not be subjected to the physical demands of this assignment.
4. She / he must be able to relate comfortably with classmates. Living quarters in a trailer are close and privacy is minimal; therefore, students cannot elect this experience if they have any preconceived antagonisms toward another student in the group.

5. Students must be willing and able to learn the variety of skills they are expected to perform, such as making a satisfactory home visit, taking a nursing history, doing an infant appraisal, giving immunization, relating to teachers on school health problems, and being amenable to taking night and weekend calls on rotation. (These are a few examples.)

Few organized rural health services require their staff to make emergency home calls or emergency clinic calls at night. Many health departments, however, are conducting night clinics to reach their working population. It is believed by the staff that when medical students are on call, it is a learning opportunity for the nurse-student to be on hand as part of the team. Moreover, students need to learn now about the changing hours of service in public health.

It is advantageous—even prerequisite—that the student (or any nurse) learn about the mores, the customs, and the language of the people in a rural county. Professional conversation becomes words of one syllable; explanations of medications or treatments are accompanied with demonstration when appropriate and are frequently repetitious. There may also be need for follow-up, either in the home or during a return clinic appointment. Many families need to be reeducated in regard to medications or health practices. Strangely enough, one of the most difficult procedures to teach is proper hand-washing before doing self-treatment in the home. Neglect of hand-washing is often not recognized as related to the transmission of pathogens in a rural atmosphere. This is only *one* aspect of the great need for health education and the prevention of illness—all of which must be discussed in simple terms, sometimes using folk language.

In the past in many rural counties, when there were two or three public health nurses, they were expected to make home visits to take blood pressure once a month, to transport a bottle of insulin, or to call just to see how the family was feeling. This is exactly what nurses used to do and the people became accustomed to *this kind* of service. It is costly use of the nurses' time, with no evaluative basis, and it did not improve the health of the community. Group health education, as has been discovered in more sophisticated zones, is one answer to better productivity and quality of care. Both students and staff nurses have difficulty, for example, getting people with diabetes mellitus together for a series of discussions about their condition. This is partly due to the enduring custom of more individualized treatment and partly due to the attitude about the condition: "It really isn't anything to be concerned about." It will take time to educate the population to respond to the group situation. Nevertheless, group therapy is an economy measure which demands implementation now.

Generally, the population is not appreciative or sensitive to the prevention of illness. Sickness is a part of life; hence it is accepted as inevitable. As one effort toward the prevention of illness, students have conducted several immunization campaigns with the result that the immune level of the population at risk has risen significantly. The immune level of a population, however, requires constant surveillance, so that immunizations cannot be a "once-every-four-years" campaign. The subject demands continuing education by the health center staff and constant availability of the immunizing material. Continuing education is not a peculiarity of immunizations. Early case findings of chronic diseases require their share of attention by modern screening devices and by personnel who are willing to do it—in this case nursing students and their faculty.

From the faculty viewpoints, the foremost purpose of this practical learning experience is to develop an awareness and concern in nursing and medical students for rural health problems and their solutions. Actual practice is one way for students to learn in a life situation, that is, treating the broken arm, the third degree burn, the lacerated hand, the myocardioinfarction, the schizophrenic individual in crisis. People in a small community experience these emergencies just as people do in metropolitan areas.

An educational experience in community nursing should have specific behavioral objectives. Briefly, the major ones are:

1. The students and faculty should provide comprehensive ambulatory care to all members of the community.
2. The milieu should be one in which nursing and medical students can learn together, as a team, about family health needs.
3. The students should live in a rural community where they get to know the people and the people get to know them. The "getting-to-know-you" part sometimes elicits a slow response from some students, but most of them begin learning to help cope with family problems evident in day-to-day existence and learning that patients are not simply a diagnosis but a reality in a social structure.
4. The students should learn to practice preventive medicine, health maintenance, and therapeutic care.

In a rural locality of limited economic and educational advantages, both faculty and students have had to learn to bridge the gap between "us" and "them." An overt effort has to be made to understand the culture and the subcultures of the population—white and nonwhite. Value systems must be identified; dual sets of values exist in all cultures, but the individual may not be conscious that he has a choice.

Learning the practice of community health in an agricultural economy means first learning to know people and how they differ from a population compacted within a city's limits. Both students and faculty members, new to the scene, must extend themselves and willingly relate person-to-person with the people they are serving. As we have discovered in the United States in our foreign aid programs, we cannot rush in and impose our systems on a different culture; so, accordingly, we cannot do it in our own country. First, the trust of the people must be established; second, a service which can be accepted by the population served must be implemented; third, the service must provide theoretical and practical learning opportunities for the faculty and students; fourth, there must be a coordinated continuing health plan which is directly related to the preventive and therapeutic services offered to the recipients of care.

EDUCATION PROBLEMS AND ADVANTAGES
OF THE RURAL HEALTH CENTER AS A
SETTING FOR NURSING EDUCATION

As education of the health-related professions tends to be located in teaching hospitals and medical centers, which in turn tend to be in urban areas, the geographical disparity becomes a transportation concern for students and faculty. The Lafayette County Health Center, a distance of sixty-three miles to the northwest, is the equivalent of three hours driving time, round trip, from Gainesville. When students are enrolled in six hours of theory courses on campus concurrently with their laboratory practice located sixty-three miles away, this presents a travel problem of some magnitude. The faculty must also travel the distance to spend individual and group time with students during the academic quarter, and they also have academic responsibilities including nursing practice at the medical center.

At the onset of this program, each of two faculty members of the community nursing section stayed two and one-half days a week, successively, in Lafayette County. When this became unrealistic from a standpoint of time and cost, the situation was relieved somewhat by the adaptation of a nurse internship appointment, a clerkship appointment, and a nurse resident appointment during various quarters. Although these additional personnel required extra time from a faculty member, this was offset by the teaching and supervision these advanced students could contribute in the instructor's absence. All of these advanced students had had one quarter (10 weeks) of practice as senior nursing students, so they were knowledgeable about routines and deviations from routines. Descriptions of the clerkship, internship, and residency were composed so that each advanced student knew the philosophy, objectives, expectations, assignments, and mutual goals of the appointment.

In the medical center the library is rich in references. For community health courses the extensive bibliography is placed on the reserve shelf. The students who are sixty-three miles from the campus library must have access to the same books as those who remain at home. Consequently, there is a duplication of references in each location.

Duplication of texts, periodicals, and articles is costly. Major textbooks have been purchased by the College of Nursing. Articles from professional journals, which are used profusely, are xeroxed so they are available at both sites. Though there must be an accounting for this expense, it is a lesser expenditure than supplying an annual journal subscription. Faculty have lent personal copies to the reference shelves; they have also contributed duplicated copies, reflecting the interest of the faculty in the course.

When planning a practicum which will have several locations, it is mandatory that the cost of the bibliography be ascertained and then multiplied by the number of units of experience. A precise number of dollars cannot be expressed here, because references are related to content and to the faculty members' favoritism. These variables and others preclude a statement of actual cost.

While the students are living in Mayo during the week, they do not have easy access to lectures, programs, theatricals, or special social events. Their major socialization is within the student group. Some students develop a relationship with the town people, but this is, of necessity, transient.

The understanding which evolves from the close association of medical and nursing students proves to be rewarding to both. They

find out that each is human and they have many goals in common
—the commonest one being improvement of patient care, and next,
the improvement of care delivery to families at a time when it is
needed.

The students must have the tools for their trade and the appropriate place to use them. They must also have living quarters which
are safe and provide a healthful environment. In a rural region this
provision is as much the responsibility of the educator as of the
administrator. Although individual students are expected to keep
their home away from home clean, they are not expected to mend
broken doors, repair television sets, or re-upholster furniture. The
instructor does have a responsibility to know the condition of the
living quarters, since the students not only live there but also use it as
their study area.

The students who volunteer for this service, more strenuous
mentally and physically (compared to the rest of the class who are
stationed in a local, urban health department that does not deviate
greatly from traditional services), seem to value highly this assignment. The reasons they give have an interesting consistency:

This is an opportunity to perfect my technical skills and to
relate to different people than I have ever known.

I chose this because I knew I could learn some different
procedures in a different environment but I would also be able to
adapt them after I graduate.

It seemed to me this would broaden my nursing education and
that I would feel more confident when I am employed as a
graduate nurse.

I thought this would be educationally exciting. It would demand more of me than I have had to give so far; and I want to be
sure of myself with technical procedures as well as interpersonal
relationships.

Other students have told me what a great experience this is. I
want to learn everything I can while I am here in Mayo. This will
help me when I go into the Navy Nurse Corps.

My expectations in nursing have been met for the most part,
but I would like to have a study area where I could be alone and
concentrate.

I feel I have not had enough experience in school health

programs. It doesn't seem to me that the school is really interested in the prevention of illness.

There is a real opportunity for learning that builds confidence in nursing procedures; however, the travel back and forth to Gainesville is tiring and such a waste of time.

Though the preparation of nurse practitioners in *primary health care* is not at this time an objective of this learning laboratory, it is natural for at least one phase of such a curriculum. Space does not allow for elaboration on the potential. If others reading this book are planning for primary health care programs, consideration might be given to the use of a similar facility.

These few quotations are a striking example of the reactions expressed by the seventy-six students who have had their practicum in the Lafayette County Health Center, including activities in the clinic, community health education projects, and home visits.

Students have had a unique experience which probably could be duplicated only in another rural region. They either collaborate on, or individually write, an article for the local newspaper (published once a week) on a current topic of disease, prevention of disease, a health center activity such as glaucoma screening, or a nursing student activity in the schools. The articles *are* published and are actually welcomed by the editor. This makes writing worthwhile for the student. She is not writing just another paper for the instructor; she is writing something original for the public to read. This can be even more satisfying, educationally, than a letter grade which attaches a label of approval of the student's ingenuity in manipulating words for the instructor's satisfaction. Students enjoy this newspaper assignment, because they see themselves in print, and that print may have a favorable effect on the life of the reader.

The Florida Division of Health has been actively interested in the project since its inception. It has demonstrated an extraordinary interest in the evolution of the educational aspects of nursing student education. Students have continuous opportunity to work with consultants from the various sections of the state agency, not only in a consulting relationship but also in program planning and the activation of the plan. For example, students determined, from the known cases of diabetes mellitus, that a county-wide screening program should be carried out. The specialized consultant from the state agency has worked closely with the students on preplanning and has assisted during the actual screening process. Students have used their own creativity in publicizing the purpose, date, time, and place. They have taken into consideration availability of the screening center for all people in the county and set up satellite stations to reach the small communities which are distant from the hub of major activity. This opportunity for students to learn (through personal contact) to use the resources at the state level is a distinct advantage which cannot be duplicated in most nursing curricula for public health. It does not occur as often for the students (in the course) who are having their laboratory in Alachua County in a traditional health department setting.

Before students commit themselves to the assignment of community health nursing in a rural area, they are informed that they must be willing to give of themselves in all phases of nursing practice, that the use of self in helping patients to meet needs is basic in all nursing activities. Few students have failed to meet this criterion.

Summarizing the evolution of this program points up financial, social, and educational considerations for students *particularly* and, to some extent, for the faculty.

Financial. The College of Nursing pays housing expenses for the students; otherwise students would be paying for residence accommodations in Gainesville as well as in Mayo. Students underwrite all of their travel (mileage) intra- and intercounty. Although this is explained explicitly during orientation, the hard facts become realistic only when the student is confronted with the situation. This would be an unfair charge against a student's educational budget. Food, of course, has to be purchased wherever one lives. Nevertheless, students accept these stipulations without complaints. They feel the experience is worth the price.

Social. Learning through socialization with medical students, resident physicians, attending physicians, nursing faculty, and state-wide consultants has proved to be an enriching experience for nursing students. Within the confines of a teaching hospital, nursing students may not have the opportunity to relate directly to the focus of a family health problem. Why should they? The nursing students often are not an invited participant in a patient-centered conference in the teaching hospital.

In the interdependency situation of the rural satellite, there is more time and inclination to include the nursing student in the analysis and planning for long-range patient care. The service situation is less formal and more obviously professionally interdependent than is the protocol of a teaching hospital.

Educational. It is the responsibility of public health nursing to bring into focus the accumulated learning from other clinical areas for application to families and groups. Many students say, "I am applying much of what I have learned in the other clinical areas to my practice in community health nursing." (That this is our singular experience may be due to our present curriculum. Other colleges of nursing will likely encounter other responses from students.) Students in a baccalaureate program are generalists in community health nursing, so the expectation of applying basic knowledge is normal in their development in this clinical area.

RELATIONSHIP BETWEEN THE NURSE AND OTHER HEALTH PERSONNEL IN A RURAL SETTING

Compatibility cannot be legislated, but it is something to which people can pledge allegiance. It is a prime requisite for selection to be part of the Lafayette County group; it is equally requisite that an atmosphere of compatibility be maintained throughout the rotation. A few errors have been made in the selection of individuals for the role of nursing student in a rural region. Of a total of 76 students, 3 proved to be misfits in some interpersonal relationships—principally with fellow nursing students as they manifested idiosyncratic behavior. Students who elect this experience usually have a genuine curiosity for how the other half lives, so they are willing to adjust to the native attitudes and beliefs in order that they might understand a rural point of view.

At the operational level, students have adjusted satisfactorily with the clerical personnel, all of whom are residents of the county and who can function like a city directory in addition to the tasks outlined by their job descriptions. One of the most helpful functions which the clerks perform is giving directions to a home located "five miles west on road 22; turn left at the first dirt road—there is an abandoned shack on that corner; turn right at the next dirt road; it is the third house on the left." Since records do not come with travel directions automatically recorded in a rural area, it is greatly timesaving to have clerks who can direct us correctly to our destinations, particularly in the outlying areas where dirt roads form the passageway and road signs are sparse.

The establishment of workable and recreational relationships with medical students and the resident is one of the objectives of the assignment. There is an aura of "We're all in this together, so we might as well get along with each other," and get along they do. All students usually share their evening meal together. The girls take turns cooking and shopping; the men sometimes take their turn at washing dishes. Occasionally, there is a medical student who is willing to exchange his white coat for an apron, and he will whip up his culinary masterpiece, such as spaghetti or spareribs.

All students are often invited by local groups to a Suwannee River catfish fry, replete with hush puppies. This is usually a gala event, and there is little food left over for hushing the puppies. The fish fry is one more opportunity for the students to talk informally —but none the less importantly—with the citizenry of the county.

Perhaps one of the most accurate indicators of the value of students to other employed personnel in the operation is their absence between academic quarters. "Now let's see, when did you say the nursing students are coming back? When does the next quarter begin?" Everyone feels (and expresses) a loss during their absence, and everyone rejoices when they are present, naturally, because the students assume a generous portion of the clinic caseload as well as the home-visit caseload. When there are no nursing students between quarters, the burden of service falls upon the clerical personnel to escort patients into examining rooms and to assist with a pelvic examination on occasion. The staff nurse (hired by the health department) must devote more of her time to the clinic, where twenty-five to thirty-five patients may be seen in a day.

Though the actual dimensions of space are discretely described and the configuration of this rural land is only 553 square miles, there are a variety of people to whom students must adjust. They find it a challenge, not a bore. They make friends only to find at the end of the quarter that "parting is such sweet sorrow." Students do more giving than receiving, which gives them a sense of usefulness quite different from anything they have known before—if one is to accept their declarations. They discover a colleague relationship between medicine and nursing which, heretofore, has been a theory and, in this situation, becomes a reality. Students no longer stand in awe of attending physicians; they communicate with them as peers, because the physician opens the door for this kind of thought exchange.

Students attend local services of worship, and they are welcomed as though they were oldtimers. These relationships may sound idealistic, but they are true, and they will withstand the closest scrutiny by anyone who doubts their authenticity.

At the onset of this program, the need to orient students for personal adjustment to the population and the environment was considered by faculty members to be of prime importance. For nursing students, a preorientation session is held in Gainesville. The second orientation is held in the Lafayette County Health Center and the town of Mayo.

Students are introduced to families in the community; in many instances, they introduce themselves. Friendliness is the key word, and it pays rich dividends in productive personal relationships.

It is agreed by the staff that preparation of the student must be a positive yet truthful one. Students get the message and are able to transmit it in action which contributes to a smooth-running project.

Unique Dimensions of the Nurse-Patient Relationship in a Rural Community

The difference between public health nursing in the urban site and on a rural scene is simple to explain. The nurse is one of many in the ghetto; her identity may be lost in the fluctuating crowd. Even in urbania the uniform is no longer distinctive or given preferential courtesy. In the rural area the nurse is seen; she is distinguished by the image of the county nurse, conceived by the population, based on their experiences with various county nurses in the past. The nurse is a kind, helpful person who assists them to cope with their sickness and health needs. She is an accepted part of the social environment. A full-time public health nurse employed with the health department may fulfill this role model to the satisfaction of the community, but the people still recognize that the nursing students do something for them which is highly individualized in relation to certain families. They feel, consequently, that they receive a more extensive service than they would enjoy were it not for nursing students. Usually, whenever there are students, the services are multiplied by the sheer numbers of personnel.

The evolving relationships between family and nurse in a rural climate are best illustrated by citing actual family studies which have been done by staff or student nurses. The following is excerpted from a student's critical analysis of a home visit.

The purposes of the visit were (1) to check Mrs. A.'s eyes; (2) to gather data on Christopher's and Edward's visual problems; (3) to review low salt diet.

A home visit was the only way in which these three purposes could be carried out at one time in an economical way. Additional data were also needed. Mention was made that the boy had had "visual problems." The only action recorded in the history was that Edward had been moved to the front row in school. It was also necessary to find out what medical follow-up Edward was receiving for his kidney infection.

To supplement my teaching of a low sodium diet, I took a copy of a sample meal plan which listed foods to be omitted and those permitted. The meal plan was discussed carefully with Mrs. A., and she indicated by responses that she understood the meaning of "low salt" in her diet.

Redness and swelling of the eyes had decreased considerably since my last visit to Mrs. A. She was not wearing sunglasses at this time; photophobia had decreased; the physician had advised that she not read or do close work until after her next appointment.

I told Mr. and Mrs. A. that I had read in the chart about Christopher's and Edward's visual problems and asked if anything had been done. Edward had been moved to the front row in school, where he could read the blackboard better. She said they had bought Christopher glasses and as a result he was not stumbling or falling over objects.

While reviewing Edward's diet with Mr. and Mrs. A., I learned they were unable to find any Lonolac milk in Mayo. I told them I would arrange with the druggist to have a supply on hand.

Though they agreed that Edward had missed a great deal of school, they stated that the physician had ordered rest and quiet play at home for another month.

The willingness with which Mr. and Mrs. A. talked with me, answered questions, and volunteered information caused me to believe that they are united in their efforts to provide good care for their children. Both ceased what they were doing when I arrived at their home and remained present during the entire interview. Neither "took over" the interview, but each contributed equally, looking to each other for agreement and clarification of questions answered. They spoke freely and openly of their need for financial assistance and seemed genuinely pleased and interested when I stated that I would look into something for them (e.g., asking the druggist to stock

Lonolac, speaking to Edward's teacher, checking the dental clinic for Larry). I sensed no feeling from them of resistance to anything I said. I received no negative responses. . . .

In this case the nurse established a nonjudgmental, workable relationship with the family and interceded on their behalf to get action from such resources as the community provided. For the nurse to ask the druggist to order a special kind of milk for a child would be most unusual in a metropolis. In a rural setting it is accepted behavior.

Excerpted from another critical analysis of a student nurse relationship is the following:

> . . . Due to the distance of the Maternal Infant Care clinic from Mayo and Janet's lack of transportation, it is felt that this [MIC] medical service is not presently meeting the health needs of Janet. These health needs are more adequately being fulfilled by the services of the local county health department and its personnel in the form of home visits, with teaching and instructions given by the staff of the *local* health department.
> Janet states she had no difficulty in understanding the medical instruction given to her by the doctor and the nurse at the MIC clinic. However, she was unable to remember what instructions were given her except that she should return if she "had any problems." No explanation was given to her as to what kind of problems they were referring to. Janet states she has only seen the doctor once and he talked to her only during the physical exam. She states the nurse talked to her for a while, but she has forgotten the contents of the conversation.
> I am unable to state fairly whether or not Janet is following any health instructions given to her by the personnel of the MIC clinic. However, I am of the opinion that the major portion of the prenatal teaching that has been given to Janet has been supplied by the student who preceded me and by myself. At least there is evidence that she remembers what was taught as exemplified by her behavior. . . .

This was not intended to be a criticism by the student of another professional group but is only to emphasize that patient education must be adjusted to the individual, and communication is a reality only when the vocabulary is adjusted to the patient's frame of reference.

The X family presented a real challenge to the nurse's ability to change behavior. The nurse had to determine the family's state of readiness for each change that was accomplished. This required infinite patience as the principal character was a woman sixty-two years of age, diabetic, and an amputee.

The initial findings by the nurse after the first assessment are as follows:

A sixty-two year old white female living with her eighty year old husband. Mrs. X has known she was diabetic for five months. She is on U 90 of NPH U80 insulin daily. Patient's left leg was amputated the first of December. She spends most of her time in bed. Her sister prepares her meals; her brother gives her insulin. She does not test her own urine nor does she know anything about her diet except that she has a "diet sheet somewhere." It is 1200 C diet prescription.

The major objectives for nursing care were to assist patient to be as independent as her capacity will allow, to test urine twice daily, to interpret diet and demonstrate practical application, to teach patient to apply Ace® bandage so that stump will be protected for an eventual prosthesis, to teach patient to become mobile either by crutch, wheelchair, or walker. Other members of the family were present whenever the nurse was teaching or demonstrating one of the objectives of care.

Home visits were made according to need—sometimes once a week, sometimes twice a week. With intensive nursing care and the involvement of the family for procedures which the patient refused to carry out, such as self-administration of insulin, the following accomplishments were recorded:

1. Patient would test urine occasionally, but never in front of the nurse. The brother always rechecked the urine after the patient had done it.

2. Patient was using a walker and moving from bedroom to living room and sitting up several hours a day. This is progress from complete bed rest (of her own volition) to becoming mobile within the house.

3. Patient has not mastered the application of the Ace bandage, through no fault of her own. She has tried. Bandage probably will have to be anchored to a belt around patient's waist to keep in place over the stump.

4. Food intake has improved—shows understanding of Food Exchange List and is able to select kinds and amounts of food allowable.

5. Patient is not receptive to instruction about the diabetic condition. At times she will turn her head away and look out of the window. At other times she will apparently listen to the nurse's instruction. . . . This is not unusual as many people with diabetes deny the diagnosis when it is first told them; some people never accept the diagnosis.

The nurse's insistence on bringing the family into the learning situation and the persistence of her teaching (demonstration and return demonstration) time with the family has effected some positive behavioral change in a few months. It is believed that this kind of nursing treatment must continue, if the patient is to be rehabilitated to her full capacity. It is interesting to note that other than the order for the amount of insulin, all other activities and procedures were implemented by the nurse based on her knowledge of the condition.

The unique aspects of the nurse-patient relationship in rural health care can also be described with students' personal notations from diaries which they have written during their rotation with the Lafayette County Health Center. Since these were unsigned manuscripts, the students could feel free to write candidly. Excerpts from nursing students' diaries:

1. We had our pictures taken for the Free Press. That was an experience. I wrote an article for publication in the paper about our first aid course. I made two home visits today. One was to CE, but she was not at home. I shall call on her tomorrow. I also saw JT in the west part of town. He is a diabetic who needed help with his diet. I spent 30 minutes talking with him, and then he spent about 30 minutes telling me about raising chickens. He had 24,500 day-old chicks delivered in the morning. It was quite an education.

2. I really feel it has been one of my valuable courses. I have done diabetic teaching including diet; I am doing prenatal instruction with a scared sixteen-year-old girl; I am reviewing and teaching the essentials of first aid. The sessions with the medical staff have been a real learning experience. I'm learning to set priorities and make decisions about what doctors need and want to know about patients. My relationships with them on a profes-

sional level have seen great improvement. I've been able to act professionally and, in turn, be treated professionally. I've made mistakes but have had my mistakes discussed and analyzed by others with me as never before.

3. Well, it's hard to believe that our rotation is up. I don't know how I could ever summarize my feelings about this experience, but I guess a good way to start is to say that I feel this has been one of the most, *if not the most*, profitable and enjoyable nursing experiences I have had while in school. . . . I knew I was right about Mayo ever since I first heard the idea proposed months ago and being here has only emphasized my initial feelings. . . . As far as technical skills are concerned I am glad that we had the chance to learn new ones and improve upon the ones we already had acquired. The doctors were more than helpful in this area. Confidence in the techniques of procedures gave me confidence to continue with the rest of my nursing knowledge.

4. I am gaining valuable experience in the art of communication. I've learned to go slowly, be tactful, and be interested when dealing with the people in the community. I think most important of all for me is the chance I have had to be exposed to the people of a different culture. In a sense I was a sheltered child, and although I have read and heard of poverty conditions, I have never really understood them until now.

5. I made a home visit to a sixty-five-year-old male with chronic emphysema, observed his wife giving him postural drainage and was impressed that even though her hands are somewhat crippled by arthritis, she makes sure he has his postural drainage three times a day.

I made a home visit with Dr. Wells to see a man who had just come home from a VA Hospital. He had a Foley catheter inserted. His wife called us because the urine was spilling into the bed instead of the plastic bag. We discovered that one of the connector tubes was stopped. This we adjusted and explained how the catheter should function. I was angry because this might have been avoided, if a nurse in the hospital had explained to the wife the care of the catheter and how it worked.

6. Today I was in the field again and made a home visit to the B family. I was fascinated with the friendliness they showed me. Mrs. B showed me her chicken house and chickens. I'd never seen so many chickens before. It was a unique experience.

7.   I was in the clinic all day. The morning seemed to be spent drawing blood for glucose tolerance tests.

We were very busy during evening clinic. I worked with a very interesting woman who had a gross amount of hematuria. We referred her to the teaching hospital for a kidney work-up on the next day. I also worked with a most adorable fifteen-month-old baby who had a very severe cough. We didn't get out of clinic until 11:45 P.M.

8.   This is the last day of our rotation. We are all going to the Rotary Club luncheon. I am looking forward to it.

I would not trade my Mayo experience for anything. It definitely has been one of the highlights of my four years at the university. I never have been able to work so closely with medical students and other professional personnel as I have here. The people [meaning townspeople] have been fantastic. I really am sad to have to leave them.

9.   The morning and afternoon was spent in the schools. It seemed scary to me at first thinking I was responsible for taking care of the children and deciding which ones should see a doctor in the clinic. After I began to work though, my fears soon began to fade. These children are remarkable. Some of them were so talkative and others so quiet, they will say something only if urged. Each one is unique. A boy came in with chicken pox. He was referred to the clinic. Many of the children had scratches and bruises which were treated topically. A number of them had stomachaches from not having had breakfast to eat. It seems to me there is a great need for better basic health education in the schools.

10. At 8:30 this morning a man was brought into the clinic in cardiac arrest. He had had a heart attack previously at home. We all worked for an hour and a half along with the resident and the medical students trying to revive him, but we couldn't.

Before going to class we stopped by to see the family of the man who had died that morning in the clinic. They seemed very grateful to us for doing what we could and stopping to see them.

The foregoing are a sample of quotations from students' evaluations. It should be obvious that they have played a major role in the development of the delivery of nursing care to a population residing in a rural community. The students have had to learn about the facts and figures of a rural region. Any graduate nurse who accepted a staff position with a local health department would have to learn the same facts and strive for the same adjustment which students have been required to do.

One student expressed this idea rather beautifully when she wrote, "I learned a lot from the doctor-nurse-patient presentations which were held daily. I only wish there were more. . . . We students have the responsibility of making the nursing part of the clinic a working entity and making ourselves, as nurses, accepted—and I think we accomplished this because we were all interested in the Mayo Project. . . . I have seen a health department through being an essential part of it, instead of being a student on the outskirts. And I have learned to know a community in a way probably impossible to duplicate again. Not only have I improved myself as a nurse but also as a person. The emphasis was on education through doing and *becoming*—and sure enough, I have done both."

Conclusion

THE PRECEDING CHAPTERS have offered readers a broad spectrum of problems and perspectives encountered in the development of a specific rural health care program. The varied viewpoints of physicians, allied health professionals, and social scientists fill these pages. The emergence of a wide range of questions and formulations is not surprising. Clinical teachers, researchers, and students bring their particular concerns to the rural health center and formulate their own conclusions concerning its significance in the community. The contributors to this volume, however, share a central, continuing experience, participation with the people of Lafayette County in developing a new resource for primary health care. The effects of that organized activity constitute the unifying theme of this book.

What were the goals underlying this joint venture between the University of Florida and the citizens of Lafayette County? The people expressed a need and a desire for more effective ways of meeting their health problems. Faculty members in the Department of Community Health and Family Medicine and teachers in the College of Nursing sought new teaching settings to introduce the student to patients in their own communities. It was apparent, in addition, that effective community service and patient care required the information and understanding derived from a continuous flow of evaluative and research studies.

How effectively are these teaching, research, and service goals being realized? The complexity of such a community project and the involvement of the editors require that judgments of success and failure be stated tentatively. Nevertheless, it is appropriate to take stock at midpoint in the first decade of the clinic's history. What has been the effect of this program on students, patients, researchers, the community, and the Colleges of Medicine and Nursing?

There are numerous indications that students experience the teaching programs at the Lafayette County Health Center as satisfying and helpful. It is the policy of the Department of Community Health and Family Medicine to institute evaluative measures at the inception of new courses. From the beginning of the clerkship programs, students and faculty have assessed this learning experience. Students have consistently given their clinical rotation weeks in Mayo high ratings. These positive expressions are not simply the result of the program's novelty. After five years of continuous clerkship teaching, we find that one-third of the students evaluate this rural health care experience as one of the best in the College of Medicine curriculum. Only a limited number of nursing students are accepted in the Lafayette County clinical program. The student demand is so great that the registration for this activity is always oversubscribed. It is difficult to know the ultimate impact of this opportunity on the later lives and practices of these future physicians and nurses. Nevertheless, teachers in subsequent courses indicate that their students often refer to insights and patient encounters derived from their Lafayette County stay, assimilating these with other clinical and basic science learnings.

The impact of these health services on the lives of Lafayette County citizens becomes increasingly apparent. They receive on-call care round-the-clock in addition to the established clinic hours. The availability of this primary care has led to a new emphasis on the prevention of illness. The school health program has been expanded. A health newsletter is circulated regularly to all county boxholders. A weight-watchers' group has been formed. The steadily increasing use of the clinic has resulted in the extension of its services. An emergency room has been added. While house calls are available, the demand for such physician activity has decreased. Correspondingly, clinic appointments have risen. This change in demand may reflect an alteration in the patients' health habits, an increasing recognition and early meeting of health needs.

The community, as well as its individual members, has felt the impact of this clinical teaching program. It is safe to say that the institution of the Lafayette County Health Center has constituted the most significant social change in this county during the last ten years. There is a marked increase in expectations and demands for comprehensive health services. One reflection of this sentiment is the fusion of county health efforts with broader primary care concerns. The traditional services provided by county health departments have been expanded to include environmental, preventive, diagnostic, and early treatment modalities. In Lafayette County, as in few others, a university professor of community health and family medicine is also the county health officer. In addition, the community displays an increasing sense of responsibility for its health care. The initial advisory committee for the Health Center is evolving into the Lafayette County Health Trust, an appointed citizens' board bearing primary responsibility for planning and administration of a comprehensive county health program.

The providers of health care soon become cognizant that they are shaped in the patient care setting as fully as their patients are. The encounter with this rural county reaches through students, house staff, and faculty into the corridors of the University Health Center, leaving a gradual but lasting imprint. The project has served as a base for an expanded four-county program of rural health service and education with support from the Robert Wood Johnson Foundation. The population served will increase from 3,000 to approximately 30,000. Concurrently, new networks of faculty cooperation are evolving as the university faces this increased rural health care challenge. The Departments of Medicine, Pediatrics, and Community Health and Family Medicine are planning jointly their teaching, research, and service offerings in primary care. It is not inaccurate to say that the cooperative effort of these university and rural populations has resulted in a crucial tilting of the thought and activity of a regional health education center.

This volume is evidence of the "soundings" conducted by researchers related to the Lafayette County Health Center. It is clear that such studies have merely scratched the surface of potential learnings. Much has been learned, however, of the need for carefully planned and coordinated studies. The researcher must not be an isolated figure. His concerns and methods must be blended with those of other investigators in the field. Rural health research is obviously a team effort in the largest sense. The rural citizen must also be seen as a colleague. His dignity and needs, as well as the integrity and requirements of scholarly study, must be maintained if "subject fatigue" and costly overlap of projects are to be avoided. The cooperative planning of these research efforts by investigators and citizens has made possible the continuation and expansion of this health care inquiry. It should be emphasized that any increments in understanding are due to the responsiveness of the people who have permitted us to share their problems and aspirations.

THE EDITORS

Bibliography

BANKS, S.A.; Murphree, Alice H.; and Reynolds, R. C. 1973. The community health clerkship: Evaluation of a program. *J. Med. Educ.* 48:560–64.

BERKI, S. E., and Heston, A. W. 1972. Introduction. *Ann. Am. Acad. Pol. Soc. Sci.* 399:ix.

BERNSTEIN, Basil. 1964. Aspects of language and learning in the genesis of the social process. In *Language and society: A reader in linguistics and anthropology*, ed. Dill Homes. New York: Harper & Row.

BRADY, P. G., and Reynolds, R. C. 1973. Rural medical practice: Computer-assisted method to study primary health care. *Postgrad. Med.* 51:249–53.

DiCANIO, Margaret B. 1971. Bilateral consensus in doctor-patient transactions. Ph.D. dissertation, University of Florida.

DOHRENWEND, B. P., and Dohrenwend, B. S. 1969. *Social status and psychological disorder: A causal inquiry*. New York: Wiley Interscience.

FLEXNER, Abraham. 1925. *Medical education: A comparative study*. New York: Macmillan Co.

FREEMAN, R. B. 1957. *Public health nursing practice*. Philadelphia: W. B. Saunders Co.

GOLDFARB, A.; Moses, L. E.; and Downing, J. J. 1967*a*. Reliability of psychiatrists' ratings in community case finding. *Am. J. Pub. Health* 57:94–106.

GOLDFARB, A.; Moses, L. E.; Downing, J. J.; and Leighton, D. C. 1967*b*. Reliability of newly trained raters in community case finding. *Am. J. Pub. Health* 57:2149–57.

GROTJAHN, Martin. 1970. Psychiatric consultations for psychiatrists. *Mental Health Dig.* 2:49–52.

HANLON, J. J. 1960. *Principles of public health administration*. St. Louis: C. V. Mosby Co.

HARRIS, L. 1968. Living sick: How the poor view their health. In *A Blue Cross report on the health problems of the poor*. Chicago: Blue Cross Assoc.

HENRY, R. A. 1972. Use of physician's assistants in Gilchrist County, Florida. *Health Services Reports* 87:687–92.

HERMAN, M. W. 1972. The poor: Their medical needs and health services. *Ann. Am. Acad. Pol. Soc. Sci.* 399:12–21.

HISCOCK, I. V. 1950. *Community health organization*. New York: Commonwealth Fund.

JONES, B., ed. 1970. *The health of Americans*. Englewood Cliffs, N.J.: Prentice-Hall.

Koos, Earl L. 1954. *The health of Regionville: What people thought and did about it*. New York: Columbia University Press.

Last, J. M., and White, K. L. 1969. The content of medical care in primary practice. *Med. Care* 7:41–48.

Leighton, D. C.; Harding, J. S.; Macklin, D. B.; MacMillan, A. M.; and Leighton, A. H. 1963. *The character of danger: Psychiatric symptoms in selected communities*. New York: Basic Books.

Lewis, C., and Resnih, B. 1967. Nurse clinics and progressive ambulatory patient care. *N. Engl. J. Med.* 277:236–41.

Ley, P., and Spelman, M. S. 1967. *Communicating with a patient*. St. Louis: Warren H. Green.

Long, R. C., ed. 1970. *A report on the health care of the poor*. Chicago: American Medical Assoc.

MacMillan, A. M. 1957. The health opinion survey: Technique for estimating prevalence of psychoneurotic and related types of disorder in communities. *Psychol. Rep.* 3:325–39.

Mead, G. H. 1934. *Mind, self, and society*. Chicago: University of Chicago Press.

Mechanic, D. 1972. Human problems and the organization of health care. *Ann. Am. Acad. Pol. Soc. Sci.* 399:1–11.

Moses, L. E.; Goldfarb, A.; Glock, C. Y.; Stark, R. W.; and Eaton, M. L. 1971. A validity study using the Leighton instrument. *Am. J. Pub. Health* 61:1785–93.

Murphree, Alice H. 1965a. *The health, resources, and practices of a rural county*. Mimeographed monograph, Division of Behavioral Sciences, Department of Psychiatry, College of Medicine, University of Florida.

Murphree, Alice H. 1965b. Folk medicine in Florida: Remedies using plants. *Fla. Anthropol.* 18:175–85.

Murphree, Alice H. 1968. A functional analysis of southern folk beliefs concerning birth. *Am. J. Obstet. Gynecol.* 102:125–34.

Murphree, Alice H., and Barrow, Mark V. 1970. Physician dependence, self-treatment practices, and folk remedies in a rural area. *South. Med. J.* 63:403–8.

Murphree, Alice H., and Barrow, Mark V. 1972. Folk medicine in Florida. *J. Fla. Med. Assoc.* 59:33–36.

National Center for Health Statistics. 1970. *Selected symptoms of psychological distress*. Ser. 9, no. 37.

Peterson, M. L. 1971. The first year in Colombia: Assessments of low hospitalization rate and high office use. *Johns Hopkins Med. J.* 128:15–23.

Reynolds, Richard C., and Cluff, Leighton E. 1971. The medical school and the health of the community: Programs developing at the University of Florida. *Am. J. Pub. Health* 61:1196–1207.

Schwab, J. J., and Warheit, G. J. 1972. Evaluating southern mental health needs and services: A preliminary report. *J. Fla. Med. Assoc.* 59:17–20.

Schwab, J. J.; McGinnis, N. H.; and Warheit, G. J. 1970. Toward a social psychiatric definition of impairment. *Br. J. Soc. Psychiatry*. Vol. 4.

Shaw, Marvin, and Costanzo, Philip R. 1970. *Theories of social psychology*. New York: McGraw-Hill Book Co.

Silver, H. K.; Ford, L. E.; and Day, L. R. 1968. The pediatric nurse practitioner program: Expanding the role of the nurse to provide increased health care for children. *JAMA* 204:298–302.

Sloan, F. A.; Clerckner, J. E.; and Wayne, J. B. 1973. Survey of north central Florida family physicians. *Fla. Fam. Phys.* 23:11–16.

Smith, Alfred G., ed. 1966. *Communication and culture: Readings in the codes of human interaction*. New York: Holt, Rinehart & Winston.

Steinman, D. 1970. Health in rural poverty: Some lessons in theory and from experience. *Am. J. Pub. Health* 60:1813–23.

UNITED STATES Department of Commerce, Bureau of Census. 1970. *Census of population: General population characteristics: Florida*. Washington.

UNITED STATES Department of Commerce, Bureau of Census. 1972. *Statistical abstract of the United States*. Washington.

UNITED STATES Department of Health, Education, and Welfare. 1971. *The economic and social conditions of rural America in the 1970's: Impact of the Department of Health, Education, and Welfare programs on non-metropolitan areas*. Washington: USGPO.

UNITED STATES Department of Health, Education, and Welfare. 1972. *Health service use: National trends and variations*. HEW Pub. no. HSM 73 3004. Washington.

UNITED STATES. President's National Advisory Committee on Poverty. 1968. *Rural poverty in the United States*. Washington: USGPO.

WARHEIT, G. J., and Hampton, A. S. 1971. *An evaluation of health care in Lake and Sumter counties, Florida*. Gainesville: Departments of Sociology and Psychiatry, University of Florida.

WARHEIT, G. J.; Holzer, C. E.; and Schwab, J. J. 1973. An analysis of social class and racial differences in depressive symptomatology: A community study. *J. Health Soc. Behavior* 14:291–99.